A₂Z in ER

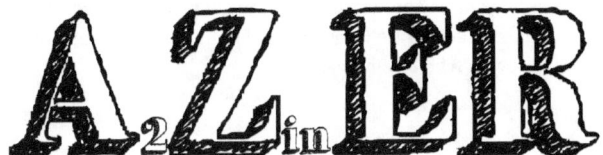

The Clinical Guide in the Emergency Room

Part 2
Clinical Classifications and Scores

First edition
2019

Mina Azer
M.B.B.Ch, Master of Surgery

Copyright © 2019 Mina Azer
All rights reserved. This book or any portion thereof may not be reproduced or used in any manner whatsoever without the express written permission of the author except for the use of brief quotations in a book review or scholarly journal.

First edition: 2019

First Printing: April 2019

ISBN-13: 9781092927062
Imprint: Independently published

Although every possible effort was made to ensure the accuracy of the information presented in this book, we cannot guarantee the absence of human error. It is also worth mentioning that we refuse to bear any moral or legal consequences by any means of false or incomplete management of patients based on information or knowledge acquired from this book. The medical field is an ever changing one, and it is the responsibility of the medical care provider to update their knowledge and skills, and to offer their patients the best possible management. One last fundamental point, medical treatment must be tailored to each individual patient. This unique management process should be the responsibility of the medical care provider along with the patient's informed consent without any predetermined management algorithms.

Acknowledgment

This work is inspired by my colleagues, both junior and senior. I was lucky enough throughout my career so far to encounter enthusiastic persons who were both eager to learn as well as pass their experience to others. This continuous process of sharing and learning was a main part of my work routine in the Gastroenterology surgical center in Mansoura University and The Egyptian Liver Institute.

I would also like to thank my colleagues in the surgery department in the Ubbo-Emmius Klinik in Norden, Germany, for being really supportive throughout the process of writing this book. I would like to thank Ibram Botros for his valuable insights and Samuel Gendy for his much appreciated technical support. Last but not least, I would like to thank Dr. Hripsime Rüstemyan and Dr. Hans-Uwe Volkers from whom I have learnt a great deal in the last three years.

This work could have never been done without the sincere support and understanding of my brave wife Mariam and my sweet angel Clara. I admit being an annoying person when consumed by a new idea. The good news is, I am done now!

Table of Contents

Chapter 1: Gallery of Common Bone Fractures   Page 09

Chapter 2: Clinical Scales and Scores

                                                     Page 55

Preface

This book is the second part of A₂ZinER© series which aims at providing a quick yet comprehensive source for medical care providers in emergency situations.

The beginning of the first night shift ever, is always a scary moment for everyone. The more experienced colleagues are already at home, and probably asleep. You are sitting in the ER or the ED waiting for the next patient, asking yourself, what would it be? A 2 cm cut wound or a perforated appendix? A mild gastroenteritis after an unfortunate fast food meal or a massive myocardial infarction? Knowing that all the possibilities are already lurking in the night outside, makes you a little bit nervous.

A₂ZinER© is the guide of the junior resident during their lonely night shifts. We assume that you have a good grasp of the basic medical knowledge. So, we won't discuss any theoretical aspects, mechanisms of action, or any other boring topics. All clutter has been ripped down leaving the very core of the addressed topics, bearing in mind the old – but still true – idiom; "common is common". In this book, you will find only the most common answers to the most common questions asked by younger colleagues.

The main idea of these books is to give you a handy tool that I wish I had during my first shifts. A concise guide to what to do and how to do it when you have no one to ask and no time to go through commercials, blocked content and false web search results to find a simple answer.

A₂ZinER© consists of 3 parts.

Part 1: Diagnostics and Investigation
A practical approach to medical diagnostic in the context of emergency situations. When to order a diagnostic test? how to perform it? and how to interpret its results? Diagnostic tests include ECG, Chest X-ray, skeletal radiology, Abdomen CT, Brain CT, Laboratory diagnostics and emergency sonography (eFAST).

Part 2: Clinical Classifications and Scores
Gallery of common bone fractures, classification and management, commonly used scoring systems and scales with a focus on emergency situations, and its interpretation according to the most recent guidelines.

Part 3: Management of emergencies
A brief and to-the-point management plan for polytrauma, nontraumatic acute chest pain, acute abdomen, and cerebral stroke. Glossary of frequently used medications (pain management, antibiotics, fluid therapy, etc..). Emergency maneuvers such as resuscitation, chest decompression, wound management, etc...

My last words to you: know the night philosophy! These could be summarized in the following points:

- ✓ Your main aim in the ER is not to miss a catastrophe more than to diagnose a rare condition.

- ✓ Stay focused on the patient's main problem. Do not get lost in the sideways.

- ✓ Learn to prioritize your actions, deal first with the problem that most likely would kill or deeply harm the patient.

- ✓ Do not perform any maneuver (diagnostic or therapeutic) during the night shift that could be postponed to the normal working hours in the next morning without harming your patient.

At last, my best wishes to my colleagues all over the world holding their position at night, guarding the human frontier against pain, suffering and death.

Mina Azer
Norden, 06ᵗʰ April 2019

Chapter 1

Gallery of Common Bone Fractures

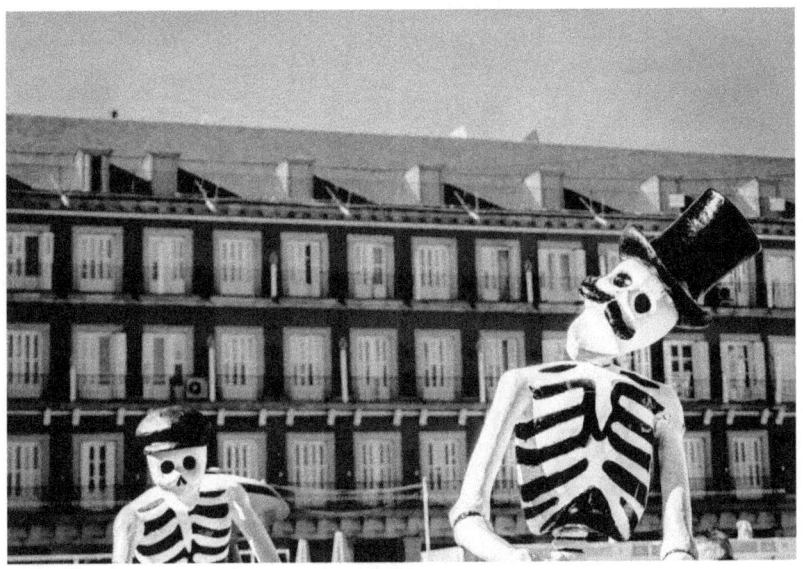

In this Chapter

Gallery of Common Bone Fractures

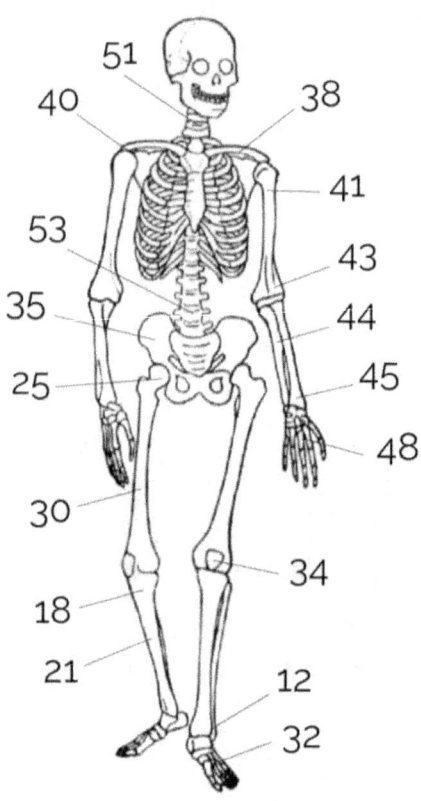

Growth Plate (Physeal) Fractures

Salter–Harris vs Aitken Classification.

Salter–Harris	Aitken	Description
I	0	fracture plane passes all the way through the growth plate, not involving bone
II	I	fracture passes across most of the growth plate and up through the metaphysis
III	II	fracture plane passes some distance along the growth plate and down through the epiphysis
IV	III	fracture plane passes directly through the metaphysis, growth plate and down through the epiphysis
V		crushing type injury does not displace the growth plate but damages it by direct compression

> Mnemonic SALTR.
> - Slipped fracture
> - Above
> - Lower
> - Through or transverse or together
> - Ruined or rammed

Salter–Harris vs Aitken classification

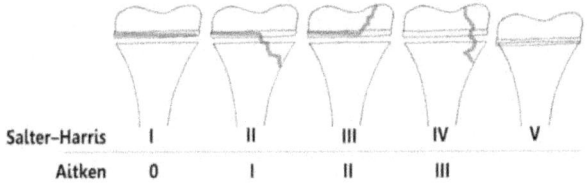

| Salter–Harris | I | II | III | IV | V |
| Aitken | 0 | I | II | III | |

Fibula

Distal fibular fracture

A fracture of the distal third of the fibula (including the lateral Malleolus). It may affect also the distal tibiofibular syndesmosis and the deltoid ligament. This fracture is usually the result of an inversion injury with or without rotation.

Weber Classification

	Weber A	Weber B	Weber C
Relation to the ankle joint	below the level of the ankle joint	At the level of the ankle joint	Above the level of the ankle joint
tibiofibular syndesmosis	intact	intact or only partially torn	disrupted
deltoid ligament	intact	intact or only partially torn	disrupted
Stability	usually stable	variable	unstable
management	conservative	variable	operative

> When examining a patient with an eversion ankle injury and clinical suspicion of medial malleolus fracture, always check the knee for proximal fibular fracture.

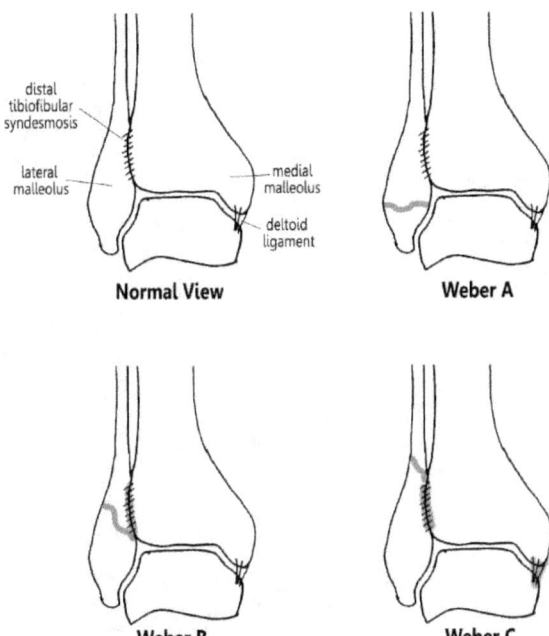

Weber classification of distal fibular fractures

Maisonneuve Fracture

A proximal spiral fibular is associated with distal tibiofibular syndesmosis rupture and the interosseous membrane. Usually associated with medial malleolus fracture or widening of the ankle joint.

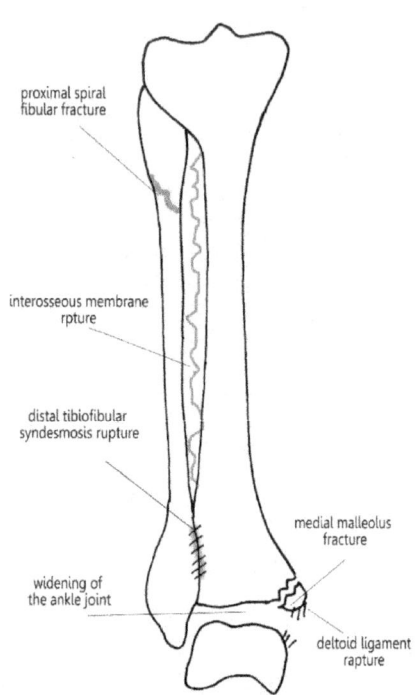

Maisonneuve fracture

Le Fort Fracture Of Ankle

This is a vertical fracture of the antero-medial part of the distal fibula with avulsion of the anterior tibiofibular ligament

Bosworth Fracture

This is a rare fracture of the distal fibula with an associated fixed posterior dislocation of the proximal fibular fragment which becomes trapped behind the posterior tibial tubercle.

Pott Fracture

Distal fibular fracture above the syndesmosis which remains intact. It is associated with deltoid ligament rupture and lateral subluxation of the talus.

Pott Fracture

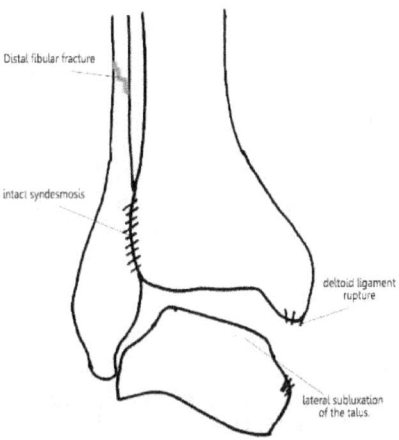

Ottawa Rules[1]

Ankle foot and knee injuries are so common that a certain clinical criteria were developed to minimize the unnecessary X-Ray investigations. X-ray is only indicated in the following conditions.

Ottawa Ankle Rule

- Pain near one or both of the malleoli PLUS *at least one* of the following:

    - Bone tenderness at the posterior edge or tip of the lateral malleolus (the distal 6 cm).
    - Bone tenderness at the posterior edge or tip of the medial malleolus (the distal 6 cm).
    - Loss of the ability of weight-bearing of the injured foot. Inability to take 4 complete steps both immediately after the injury or at the time of the examination.

Ottawa Foot Rules

- Pain at midfoot zone (tarsal area) PLUS *at least one* of the following:
    - Bone tenderness at the base of the fifth metatarsal.
    - Bone tenderness at the navicular bone.
    - Loss of the ability of weight-bearing of the injured foot. Inability to take 4 complete steps both immediately after the injury or at the time of the examination.

The Ottawa Knee Rule

- knee injury patients PLUS *at least one* of the following:

    - Age 55 or older
    - Isolated tenderness of the patella
    - Tenderness of the head of the fibula
    - Cannot flex to 90 degrees
    - Loss of the ability of weight-bearing of the injured foot. Inability to take 4 complete steps both immediately after the injury or at the time of the examination.

---

[1] http://www.theottawarules.ca

In Patients who don't meet these criteria, it is wise to advice RICE management plan with follow up in 5 to 7 days if the symptoms persisted.

> RICE management plan:
>
> Rest, Ice, Compression and Elevation.

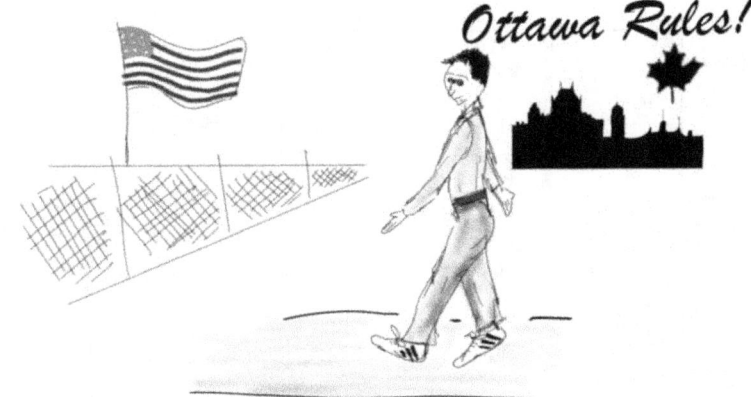

Canadian health system sucks, I am going back!

TIBIA

TIBIAL PLATEAU FRACTURE

SCHATZKER CLASSIFICATION

Type	Description
I	Wedge-shaped splitting fracture of the lateral tibial plateau.
II	Splitting and depression of the lateral tibial plateau; (type I fracture with a depressed component)
III	Pure depression of the lateral tibial plateau
IV	Medial tibial plateau fracture with a split or depressed component
V	Wedge-shaped splitting fracture of both lateral and medial tibial plateau
VI	transverse tibial metadiaphyseal fracture, along with any type of tibial plateau fracture (metaphyseal-diaphyseal discontinuity)

> Type II is by far the most common tibial plateau fracture (75% of cases). In the second place is the Type IV (20% of cases).

Schatzker classification of tibial plateau fractures

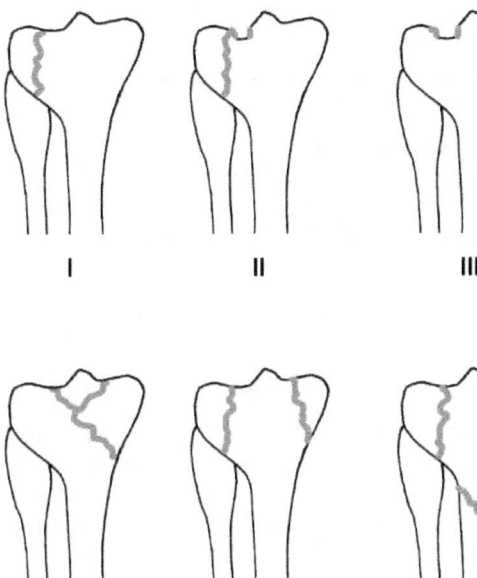

I II III

IV V VI

HOHL AND MOORE CLASSIFICATION OF PROXIMAL TIBIA FRACTURE-DISLOCATIONS

This classification is useful in fractures that couldn't be classified according to Schatzker classification or fractures associated with knee instability.

Type	Description
Type I	Coronal split fracture
Type II	Entire condylar fracture
Type III	Rim avulsion fracture of lateral plateau
Type IV	Rim compression fracture
Type V	Four-part fracture

BUMPER FRACTURE

A bumper fracture is a fracture of the lateral tibial plateau caused by a forced valgus applied to the knee. This causes the lateral part of the distal femur to compress the tibial plateau causing the fracture. Schatzker Type II.

```
The classic mechanism of injury is when
a car bumper hits the knee laterally
with foot is held stable on the ground
(weight-bearing limb).
```

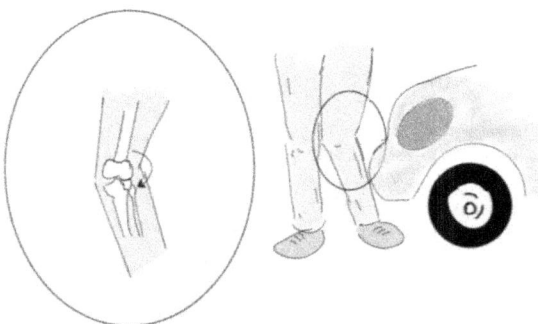

Tibia Shaft Fracture

This is a fracture of the proximal third of the tibia. It is usually associated with soft tissue injury or open wounds.

> Tibia shaft fracture is the most commonly fractured long bone in the body

Oestern and Tscherne Classification of Closed Fractuer Soft Tissue Injury

Grade	Description
0	Injuries from indirect forces with negligible soft-tissue damage
I	Superficial contusion/abrasion, simple fractures
II	Deep abrasions, muscle/skin contusion, direct trauma, impending compartment syndrome
III	Excessive skin contusion, crushed skin or destruction of muscle, subcutaneous degloving, acute compartment syndrome, and rupture of major blood vessel or nerve

Gustilo-Anderson Classification of Open Tibia Fractures

Type	Description
I	Limited periosteal stripping, clean wound < 1 cm
II	Mild to moderate periosteal stripping, wound >1 cm in length
IIIA	Significant soft tissue injury (often evidenced by a segmental fracture or comminution), significant periosteal stripping, wound usually >5cm in length, no flap required
IIIB	Significant periosteal stripping and soft tissue injury, flap required due to inadequate soft tissue coverage.
IIIC	Significant soft tissue injury (often evidenced by a segmental fracture or comminution), vascular injury requiring repair to maintain limb viability

Segond Fracture

The Segond fracture is a type of avulsion fracture (soft tissue structures tearing off bits of their bony attachment) of the lateral tibial condyle of the knee, immediately beyond the surface which articulates with the femur.

Gosselin Fracture

The Gosselin fracture is a V-shaped fracture of the distal tibia which extends into the ankle joint and fractures the tibial plafond into anterior and posterior fragments

Toddler's Fracture

Toddler's fractures or childhood accidental spiral tibial (CAST) fractures are bone fractures of the distal part of the tibia in toddlers (aged 9 months-3 years). The fracture is usually found in the distal two thirds. It occurs after low-energy trauma, sometimes with a rotational component.

Pilon fracture Plafond fracture

This is a fracture of the distal part of the tibia, involving its articular surface at the ankle joint. Pilon fractures are caused by rotational or axial forces, mostly as a result of falls from a height or motor vehicle accidents.

The Ruedi-Allgower classification is a system of categorizing pilon fractures of the distal tibia.

Type	Description
I	Non-displaced
II	Displaced but not comminuted
III	Comminuted articular surface

Tillaux fracture

A Tillaux fracture is an epiphyseal fracture (Salter–Harris type III or Aitken II) through the anterolateral aspect of the distal tibial epiphysis. It occurs in adolescents between the ages of 12 and 15. In this age the medial epiphysis is already closed before the lateral epiphysis.

Combined tibia and fibula fractures

Trimalleolar fracture

This ankle fracture is composed of 3 components: medial malleolus fracture, lateral malleolus fracture and posterior malleolus fracture. The posterior malleolus is a famous misnomer of the posterior part of the tibia, also known as Volkmann's triangle.

Bimalleolar fracture

This is an ankle fracture of both medial and lateral malleoli.

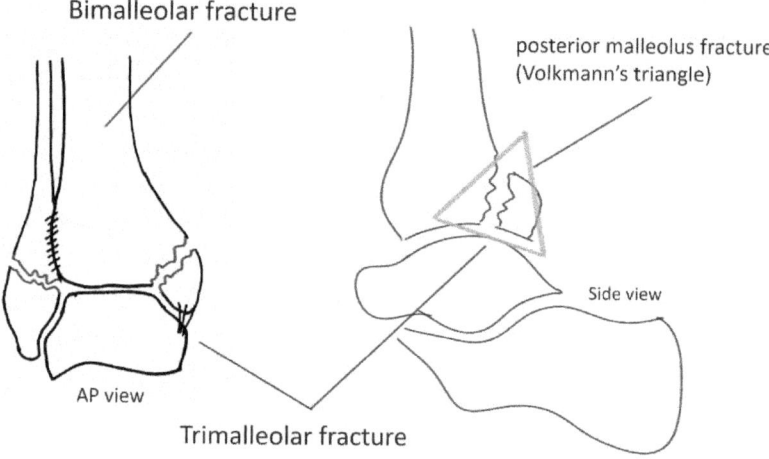

Femur

Femur head fractures

Pipkin classification
The Pipkin is a system of categorizing femoral head fractures based on the fracture pattern.

Type	Description
I	Fracture below the fovea; not involving weight-bearing surface of the head
II	Fracture above the fovea; involving weight-bearing surface of the head
III	Type I or II fracture with associated femoral neck fracture
IV	Type I or II fracture with associated acetabulum fracture

> Type III is associated with significantly increased risk of femoral head avascular necrosis.

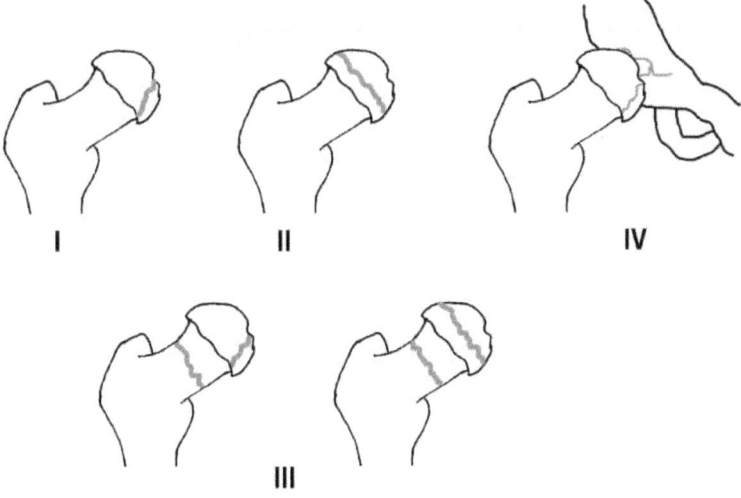

Pipkin classification

Femur neck fractures

Garden Classification
This classification is based on AP radiographs only.

Type	Description
I	Incomplete fracture or valgus impacted
II	Complete but non-displaced fracture
III	Complete, partially displaced fracture
IV	Complete, fully displaced fracture

	Simplified Version
Non-displaced	Includes Garden I and II
Displaced	Includes Garden III and IV

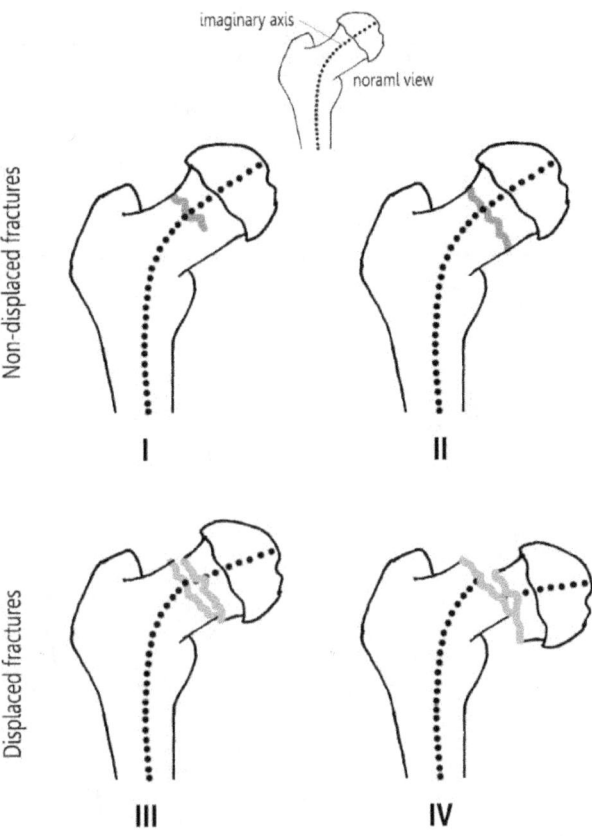

PAUWELS CLASSIFICATION
Based on vertical orientation of fracture line.

Type	Description
I	< 30 degree from horizontal
II	30 to 50 degree from horizontal
III	> 50 degree from horizontal (most unstable with highest risk of nonunion and AVN)

Pauwels Classification

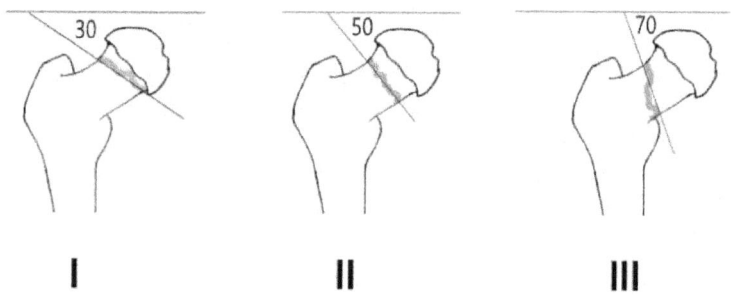

I II III

INTERTROCHANTERIC FRACTURES
EVANS-JENSEN CLASSIFICATION

Type	Description
IA	2-part non-displaced
IB	2-part displaced
IIA	3-part fracture with separate greater trochanter fragment
IIB	3-part fracture with separate lesser trochanter fragment
III	4-part fracture

MANAGEMENT OPTIONS OF PROXIMAL FEMUR FRACTURES[2]:

Some selected cases of Pauwels I fractures can be treated conservatively, otherwise surgical treatment is always recommended.

Timing of surgery: within 24 hours of admission except in unstable patients or patients under oral anticoagulant therapy.

FEMUR NECK FRACTURES
In patients with a displaced intracapsular hip fracture perform replacement arthroplasty (total hip replacement) if the patient:
- ✓ were able to walk independently out of doors with no more than the use of a stick, and
- ✓ are not cognitively impaired, and
- ✓ are medically fit for anaesthesia and the procedure.

Otherwise perform a hemiarthroplasty.

INTERTROCHANTERIC OR SUBTROCHANTERIC FRACTURES

In patients with trochanteric fractures above or including the lesser trochanter perform fixation with a sliding hip screw in preference to an intramedullary nail.

In patients with subtrochanteric fracture use an intramedullary nail.

---

[2] Hip fracture: management, Clinical guideline [CG124] – NICE guidelines. Published date: June 2011 Last updated: May 2017

Femur shaft fractures

Winquist and Hansen Classification

Type	Description
0	No comminution
I	Insignificant amount of comminution
II	Greater than 50% cortical contact
III	Less than 50% cortical contact
IV	Segmental fracture with no contact between proximal and distal fragment

Winquist and Hansen Classification

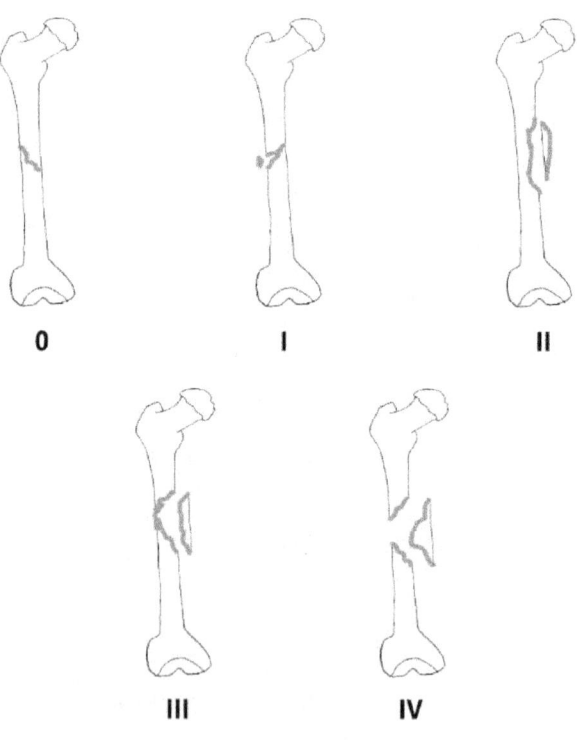

Periprosthetic fracture

Vancouver classification

Type	Subtype	Description
A	A L	Lesser trochanter
	A G	Greater trochanter
B	B1	Well-fixed prosthesis
	B2	Prosthesis loose
	B3	Prosthesis loose with poor bone stock
C		Fracture well below tip of the prosthesis

Vancouver classification

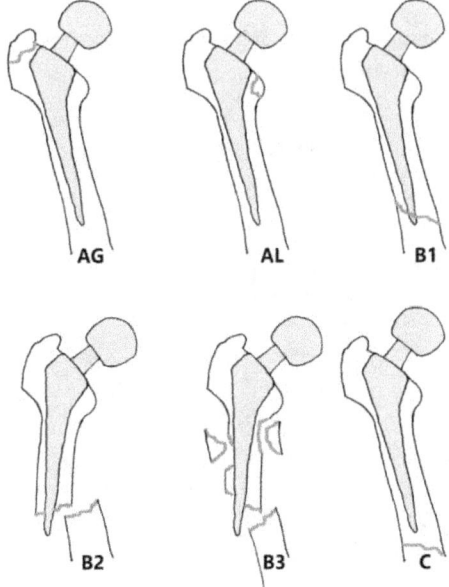

FOOT FRACTURE

LISFRANC FRACTURE

This is a fracture of the metatarsal bones associated with dislocation from the tarsus.

JONES FRACTURE

This is a between the base and the shaft of the fifth metatarsal bone.

MARCH FRACTURE

This is a fracture of the distal third of one of the metatarsals occurring because of recurrent stress. (Fatigue or stress fracture)

Foot fractures

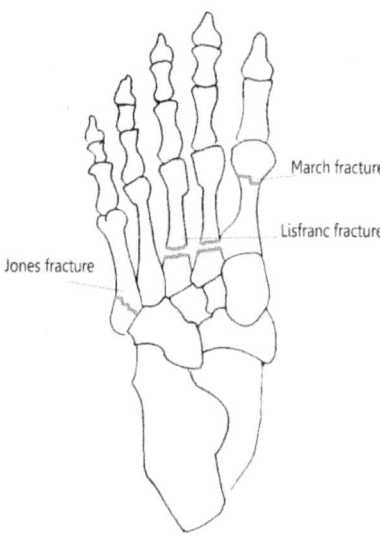

CALCANEAL FRACTURE

SANDERS CLASSIFICATION

Type	Description
I	Non-displaced posterior facet (regardless of number of fracture lines)
II	One fracture line in the posterior facet (two fragments)
III	Two fracture lines in the posterior facet (three fragments)
IV	Comminuted with more than three fracture lines in the posterior facet (four or more fragments)

Patella

Types of patellar fractures

- Non-displaced
- Transverse
- Pole or sleeve (upper or lower)
- Vertical
- Marginal
- Osteochondral
- Comminuted (stellate)

> A strong clinical hint of the patella fracture is the loss of the ability of hip flexion while maintaining the knee extension.

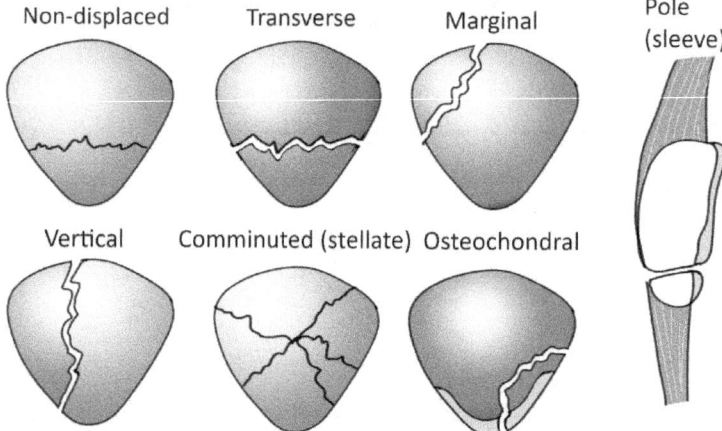

Bipartite patella (two-part patella)

A congenital finding that may be mistaken for patella fracture. It is a patella with an unfused accessory ossification center at the superolateral aspect.

Features:

- ✓ It affects 8% of population.
- ✓ Characteristic superolateral position.
- ✓ Bilateral in 50% of cases.

PELVIC FRACTURE

THE YOUNG-BURGESS CLASSIFICATION

A system of categorizing pelvic fractures based on fracture pattern, allowing the judgment on the stability of the pelvic ring.

Type	Anterior Posterior Compression APC	Lateral Compression LC	Vertical Shear VS
I	Symphysis widening < 2.5 cm	Pubic ramus fracture and ipsilateral anterior sacral ala compression fracture	Posterior and superior directed force
II	Symphysis widening > 2.5 cm. Anterior SI joint diastasis. Disruption of sacrospinous and sacrotuberous ligaments	Rami fracture and ipsilateral posterior ilium fracture dislocation	
III	SI dislocation with associated vascular injury	Ipsilateral lateral compression and contralateral APC	

TILE CLASSIFICATION

Type	Subtype	Description
A: stable	A1	fracture not involving the ring (avulsion or iliac wing fracture)
	A2	stable or minimally displaced fracture of the ring
	A3	transverse sacral fracture
B: rotationally unstable, vertically stable	B1	open book fracture
	B2	lateral compression injury
		B2-1: with anterior ring rotation/displacement through ipsilateral rami
		B2-2: with anterior ring rotation/displacement through contralateral rami
	B3	bilateral
C: rotationally and vertically unstable	C1	unilateral
		C1-1: iliac fracture
		C1-2: sacroiliac fracture-dislocation
		C1-3: sacral fracture
	C2	bilateral with one side type B and one side type C
	C3	Also associated with acetabular fracture

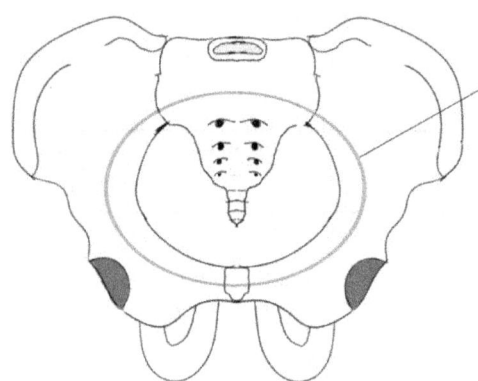

The stability of the pelvic fractures depends on the extent of damage of the pelvic ring.

Stable fracture: usually one undisplaced fracture of the pelvic.

Unstable fracture: more than one fracture of the pelvic ring at least one of then is displaced.

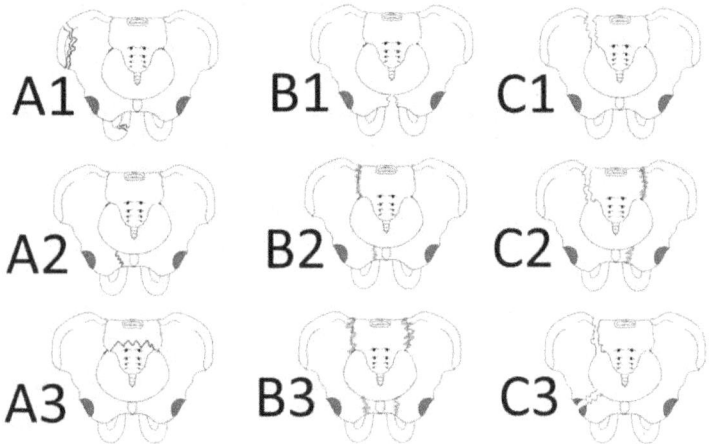

Open book fracture

One specific kind of pelvic fracture is known as an 'open book' fracture. This is often the result from a heavy impact to the pubis, a common motorcycling accident injury.

Duverney fracture

Duverney fractures are isolated pelvic fractures involving only the iliac wing. They are caused by direct trauma and are generally stable fractures.

Acetabular fracture

Tile's classification of acetabular fracture

Type	Description
I	Simple fracture, anterior or posterior wall column
II	Transverse fracture
III	T - Type fracture involving two columns
IV	Both columns fractures, floating acetabulum

Shoulder Fracture

Middle Third Clavicle Fracture

Neer's Classification

Type	Description	Treatment
Non-displaced	Less than 100% displacement	conservative treatment
Displaced	Greater than 100% displacement Nonunion rate of 4.5%	operative treatment

Lateral Third Clavicle Fractures

Neer's Classification

Type	Description
I	A minimally displaced fracture lateral to coracoclavicular ligaments with intact conoid and trapezoid ligament Stable fracture – conservative treatment
IIA	A medially displaced fracture medial to coracoclavicular ligaments with intact conoid and trapezoid ligament Unstable fracture – operative treatment
IIB	Two fracture patterns, both show signficant medial claviclular dispalcement Fracture occurs between the coracoclavicular ligaments. Conoid ligament is torn but trapezoid ligament remains intact Fracture occurs lateral to coracoclavicular ligaments with torn conoid and trapezoid ligament Unstable fracture – operative treatment
III	A minimally displaced intra-articular fracture extending to the acromioclavicular joint with intact conoid and trapezoid ligament Stable fracture – conservative treatment
IV	A laterally displaced physeal fracture with intact conoid and trapezoid ligament Stable fracture – conservative treatment
V	A medially displaced comminuted fracture with intact conoid and trapezoid ligament Unstable fracture – operative treatment

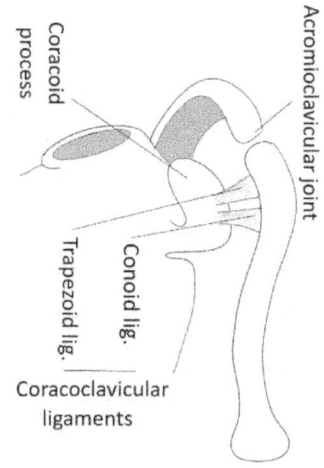

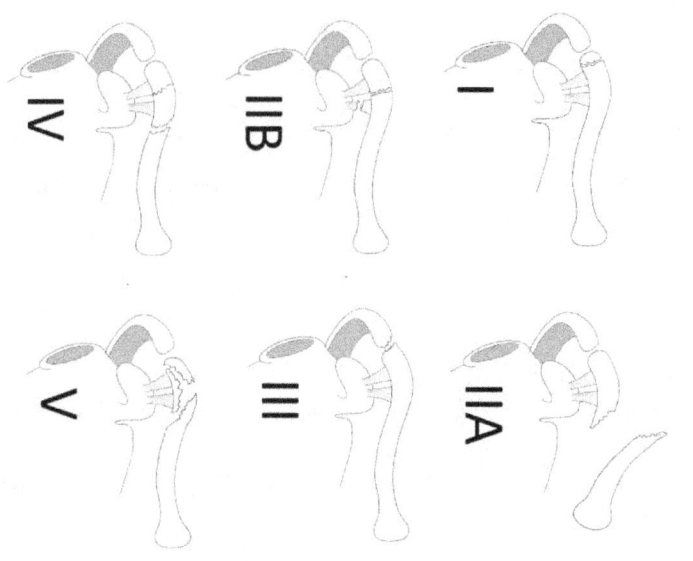

ACROMIOCLAVICULAR JOINT INJURY

TOSSY AND ROCKWOOD CLASSIFICATION
Tossy categories I to III are identical to Rockwood categories I to III. Furthermore Rockwood classification identify 3 more categories (IV to VI).

FURTHER CATEGORIES IF ROCKWOOD CLASSIFICATION

Type	I	II	III
Description	No radiological deformity	clavicle is slightly elevated	clavicle elevated above the superior border of kthe acromion
AC ligament	Mild sprain	Ruptured	Ruptured
CC ligament	Intact	Sprain	Ruptured
joint capsule	Intact	Ruptured	Ruptured
deltoid muscle	Intact	Minimally detached	Detached
trapezius muscle	Intact	Minimally detached	Detached

AC: acromioclavicular, CC: coracoclavicular.

Categories IV to VI are described as the category III with the following variations:

- ✓ **IV:** the clavicle is displaced posteriorly into the trapezius.

- ✓ **V:** the clavicle is markedly elevated where the coracoclavicular distance is more than double normal (i.e. >25 mm).

- ✓ **VI:** the clavicle is inferiorly displaced behind coracobrachialis and biceps tendon.

AC injury diagnosis

Clinically: tenderness of AC joint after a direct trauma. Piano key sign may be present.
X-Ray: the inferior borders of the lateral clavicular end and the acromion should be on the same level. If not, think of ligament injury. This can be assessed by measuring the following distances:
- Acromioclavicular (AC) distance >8 mm: AC ligament rupture
- Coracoclavicular (CC) distance >13 mm: CC ligament rupture

Humerus

Proximal Fractures

Neer's Classification

Basic concepts of Neer's classification:

In this classification the proximal humeral end is divided into 4 parts: humeral head (or the articular surface), greater tuberosity, lesser tuberosity and humeral shaft.

The surgical neck separates the shaft form the tuberosities above while the anatomical neck separates the articular surface from the tuberosities below.

A fracture is regarded as displaced if the angulation is more than 45 degrees or the 2 fragments are displaced by more than 1cm.

Type	Description	Common pattern
One-part fracture	fracture lines involve 1 to 4 parts, none of them is displaced	Surgical neck
Two-part fracture	fracture lines involve 1 to 4 parts, one of them is displaced.	surgical neck (85%)
Three-part fracture	fracture lines involve 2 to 4 parts, two of them is displaced.	displaced greater tuberosity and shaft.
Four-part fracture	fracture lines involve 3 to 4 parts, three of them is displaced	Generally rare.

> The terms one-part and two part etc. refers to the proximal humerus as a whole. In a one part fracture, in which nothing is displaced, the proximal humerus, despite being fractured, is considered as a ONE Part. On the other hand a two-part fractures means that one part is displaced (not only fractured) from the proximal humeral complex (the other Part).

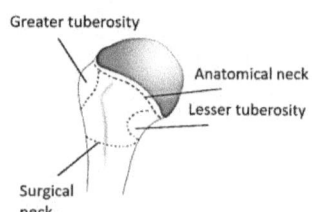

Neer I: minimally displaced fractures
Neer II: anatomical neck
Neer III: surgical neck
Neer IV: G. Tuberosity
Neer V: L. Tuberosity
Neer VI: Fracture-dislocation

	1 Part	2 Parts	3 Parts	4 Parts
I	◯			
II		◯		
III		◯		
IV		◯	◯	◯
V		◯	◯	
VI	Proximal humerus fracture combined with anterior or posterior shoulder dislocation			

Supracondylar Fracture

A supracondylar humerus fracture is a fracture of the distal humerus just above the elbow joint. This fracture is more common in children. There are 2 subtypes of this fracture according to the mechanism of injury: Extension Type (95% of cases - Hyperextension occurs during a fall onto an outstretched hand) and Flexion Type in only 5% of cases.

Gartland Classification of Extension Supracondylar Fracture

Type	Description
I	non-displaced fractures
II	angulated fractures
III	Angulated with complete separation between the 2 fragments

> Neurovascular complications (The Pink and Pulseless hand) is relatively common in supracondylar fractures due to tear, spasm or entrapment of the brachial artery.

Holstein-Lewis Fracture

This is a fracture of the distal third of the humerus resulting in entrapment of the radial nerve.

Ulna

Monteggia fracture

This is a fracture of the proximal third of the ulna with dislocation of the proximal head of the radius.

Hume fracture

The Hume fracture is an injury of the elbow comprising a fracture of the olecranon with an associated anterior dislocation of the radial head which occurs in children. It can be considered a variant of the Monteggia fracture.

Olecranon Fractures

Schatzker Classification

Type	Description
A	Simple transverse fracture
B	Impacted transverse fracture
C	Oblique fracture
D	Comminuted fracture
E	More distal fracture, extra-articular
F	Fracture-dislocation

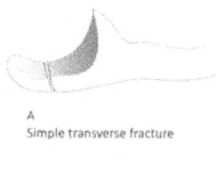
A
Simple transverse fracture

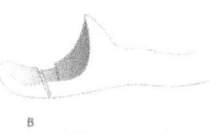
B
Impacted transverse fracture

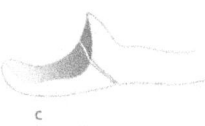
C
Oblique fracture

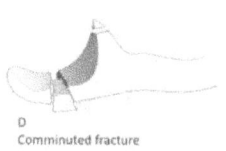
D
Comminuted fracture

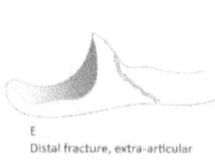
E
Distal fracture, extra-articular

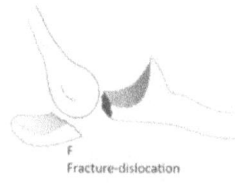
F
Fracture-dislocation

RADIUS

RADIAL HEAD FRACTURES

MASON CLASSIFICATION (MODIFIED BY HOTCHKISS AND BROBERG-MORREY)

Type	Description
I	Non-displaced or minimally displaced (<2mm), no mechanical block to rotation
II	Displaced >2mm or angulated, possible mechanical block to forearm rotation
III	Comminuted and displaced, mechanical block to motion
IV	Radial head fracture with associated elbow dislocation

> **Terrible Triad Injury of Elbow**
> - ✓ elbow dislocation (posterior)
> - ✓ radial head or neck fracture
> - ✓ coronoid fracture
>
> One of the difficult fractures to manage due to persistent instability, stiffness and arthrosis.

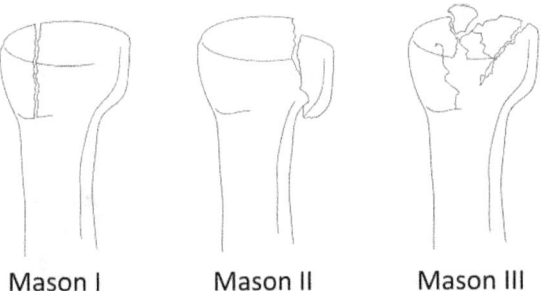

Mason I   Mason II   Mason III

Essex-Lopresti Fracture

This is a fracture of the radial head with concomitant dislocation of the distal radio-ulnar joint and disruption of the interosseous membrane.

Galeazzi Fracture

The Galeazzi fracture is a fracture of the distal third of the radius with dislocation of the distal radioulnar joint.

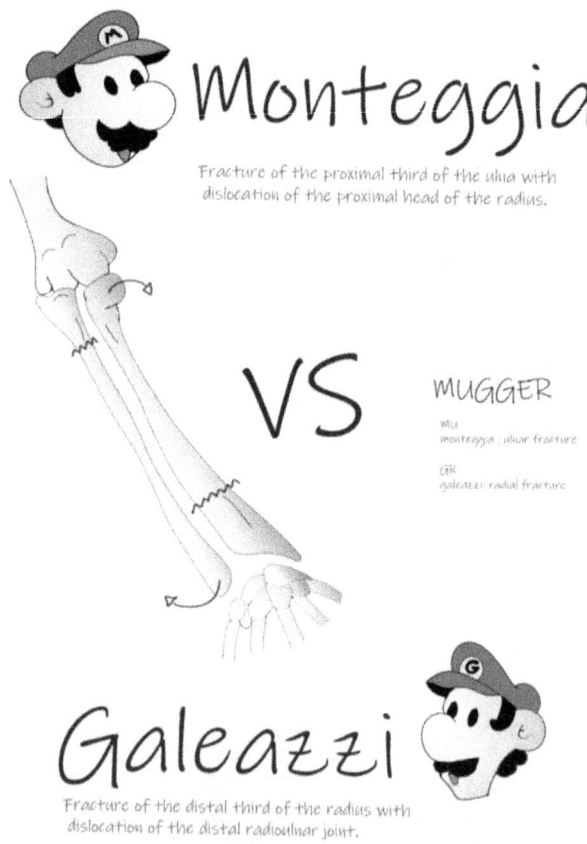

Monteggia
Fracture of the proximal third of the ulna with dislocation of the proximal head of the radius.

VS

MUGGER
MU
monteggia : ulnar fracture

GR
galeazzi : radial fracture

Galeazzi
Fracture of the distal third of the radius with dislocation of the distal radioulnar joint.

Colle's Fracture

This is the most common wrist fracture sustained in a FOOSH injury. It refers to a fracture of the distal radius with dorsal angulation and sometimes displacement of the distal fragment, producing a silver fork deformity. This term is used because the deformity resembles an upside-down dinner fork when the wrist is viewed laterally. This injury occurs most frequently in older women with osteoporosis

Frykman Classification

Type	Ulna fracture absent	Ulna fracture present
Extra articular	I	II
Intra-articular involving radiocarpal joint	III	IV
Intra articular involving distal radio-ulnar joint	V	VI
Intra articular involving both radiocarpal & distal radioulnar joints	VII	VIII

Smith's Fracture

This is similar to a Colles fracture but the distal radius is volarly displaced. These fractures typically occur in younger patients and often are associated with other wrist injuries.

Barton's Fracture

This is a variant of Colles fracture in which the distal radius is sheared off, causing proximal migration of the distal fragment and dislocation of the radiocarpal joint. A Barton fracture requires immediate orthopedic referral for surgical repair

Chauffeur Fractures Fracture

(also known as Hutchinson fractures or backfire fractures) these are intra-articular fractures of the radial styloid process. The radial styloid is within the fracture fragment, although the fragment can vary markedly in size

Hand

Scaphoid Fracture

Fracture of the scaphoid bone is characterized by tenderness and swelling of the anatomical snuffbox. Complications may include nonunion of the fracture, avascular necrosis, and arthritis.

Mayo Classification

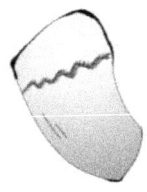 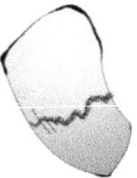 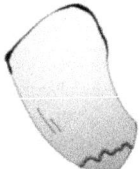

Distal Third   Middle Third   Proximal Third

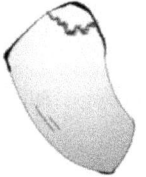 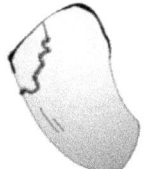

Distal Tubercle   Distal Articular Surface

Risk of avascular necrosis (AVN) depends on the location of the fracture.

- ✓ Fractures in the proximal 1/3 have a high incidence of AVN (~30%)

- ✓ Waist fractures in the middle 1/3 is the most frequent fracture site and has moderate risk of AVN.

- ✓ Fractures in the distal 1/3 are rarely complicated by AVN.

Rolando's fracture

The Rolando fracture is a comminuted intra-articular fracture through the base of the first metacarpal bone.

Bennett's fracture

Bennett fracture is a fracture of the base of the first metacarpal bone which extends into the carpometacarpal joint. This intra-articular fracture is the most common type of fracture of the thumb, and is nearly always accompanied by some degree of subluxation or dislocation of the carpometacarpal joint.

Boxer's fracture

A boxer's fracture is the break of the 5th metacarpal bones of the hand near the knuckle.

Gamekeeper's thumb fracture

(also known as skier's thumb) this is a type of injury to the ulnar collateral ligament (UCL) of the thumb. The UCL may be torn, damaged or in some cases avulsed from its insertion site into the proximal phalanx of the thumb in the vast majority (approximately 90%) of cases.

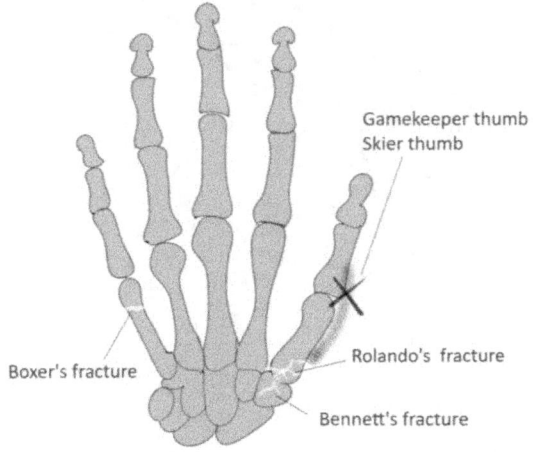

Fall onto an outstretched hand (FOOSH)

A FOOSH is an acronym of a common mechanism of injury. A fall onto an outstretched hand can cause various fractures such as:

Common Fractures	Hint
Fracture of the clavicle	Look for deformity and tenderness of the clavicula
Fracture proximal humerus	More common in older patients. A similar injury in young people may result in shoulder dislocation.
Supracondylar fracture of the humerus	More in common children
Fracture of the head and neck of the radius	Adults: head of the radius, Children: neck of the radius
Monteggia fracture-dislocation	
Galeazzi fracture-dislocation	Probably with an element of rotation.
Colles' fracture	By far the most common type
Fracture of the scaphoid	Look for tenderness of the anatomical snuffbox
Bennetts fracture	fracture of the base of the first metacarpal bone which extends into the carpometacarpal joint
Gamekeeper's thumb fracture	Ulnar collateral ligament injury

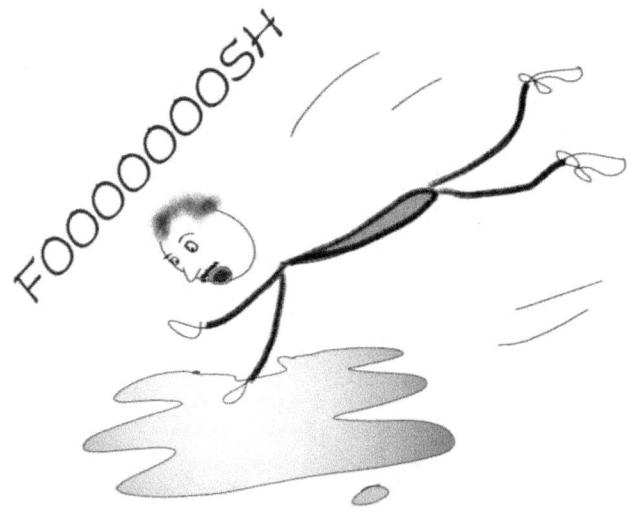

Vertebrae

Jefferson fracture

A Jefferson fracture is a bone fracture of the anterior and posterior arches of the C1 vertebra. Though it may also appear as a three- or two-part fracture. The fracture may result from an axial load on the back of the head or hyperextension of the neck (e.g. caused by diving), causing a posterior break, and may be accompanied by a break in other parts of the cervical spine.

Hangman's fracture

This is a fracture of both pedicles or pars interarticularis of the axis vertebra (C2)

Flexion teardrop fracture

A flexion teardrop fracture is a fracture of the anteroinferior aspect of a cervical vertebral body due to flexion of the spine along with vertical axial compression. A teardrop fracture is usually associated with a spinal cord injury, often a result of displacement of the posterior portion of the vertebral body into the spinal canal.

Clay-shoveler fracture

Clay-shoveler's fracture is a stable fracture through the spinous process of a vertebra occurring at any of the lower cervical or upper thoracic vertebrae, classically at C6 or C7.

FRACTURES OF THE ODONTOID PROCESS OF AXIS VERTEBRA (C2)

ANDERSON AND D'ALONZO CLASSIFICATION

Type I	rare fracture of the upper part of the odontoid peg above the level of the transverse band of the cruciform ligament usually considered stable
Type II	most common fracture at the base of the odontoid below the level of the transverse band of the cruciform ligament unstable
Type III	fracture through the odontoid and into the lateral masses of C2 relatively stable if not excessively displaced best prognosis for healing because of the larger surface area of the fracture

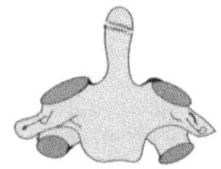 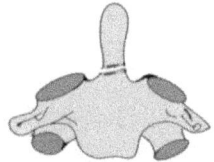 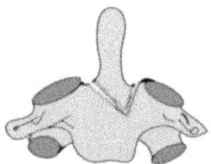

Type I   Type II   Type III

THORACOLUMBAR SPINAL FRACTURES

THREE COLUMN CONCEPT OF THORACOLUMBAR SPINAL FRACTURES
DENIS CLASSIFICATION

Denis divided the vertebral column into 3 vertical parallel columns based on biomechanical studies related to stability following traumatic injury. The fracture is considered unstable when it affects 2 adjacent columns. (i.e. anterior and middle column, middle and posterior column or the three columns).

Anterior column (AC)	Middle column (MC)	Posterior column (PC)
anterior longitudinal ligament (ALL)	posterior one-third of the vertebral body (VB)	everything posterior to the (PLL)
anterior two-thirds of the vertebral body (VB)	posterior one-third of the intervertebral disc (IVD)	pedicles (P)
anterior two-thirds of the intervertebral disc (IVD)	posterior longitudinal ligament (PLL)	facet joints (FJ)
		ligamentum flavum (LF)
		Interspinous ligament (ISL)
		Supraspinous ligament (SSL)

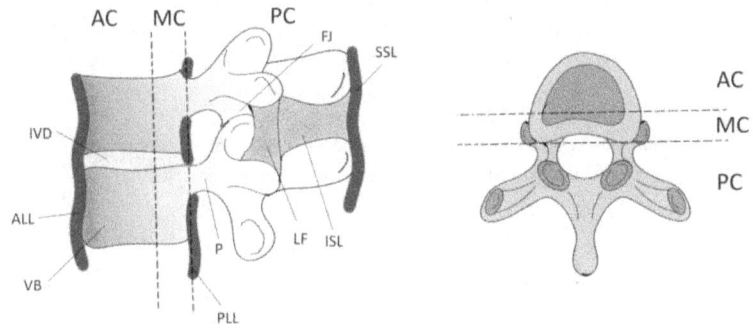

BURST FRACTURE

A burst fracture is a type of traumatic spinal injury in which a vertebra breaks from a high-energy axial load (e.g., traffic collisions or falls from a great height or high speed, and some kinds of seizures), with shards of vertebra penetrating surrounding tissues and sometimes the spinal canal. This an unstable fracture affecting the 3 columns.

COMPRESSION FRACTURE

A compression fracture is a collapse of a vertebra. It may be due to trauma or due to a weakening of the vertebra (compare with burst fracture). This weakening is seen in patients with osteoporosis or osteogenesis imperfecta, lytic lesions from metastatic or primary tumors, or infection. In healthy patients it is most often seen in individuals suffering extreme vertical shocks, such as ejecting from an ejection seat.

CHANCE FRACTURE

A Chance fracture is a flexion injury of the spine. It consists of a tension-failure injury to the anterior column of the vertebral body and a transverse fracture through the posterior elements of the vertebra and the posterior portion of the vertebral body. It is caused by violent forward flexion, causing distraction injury to the posterior elements.

The most common site at which Chance fractures occur is the thoracolumbar junction (T12-L2). Up to 50% of Chance fractures have associated intraabdominal injuries.

HOLDSWORTH FRACTURE

This is an unstable fracture dislocation of the thoraco lumbar junction of the spine. The injury comprises a fracture through a vertebral body, rupture of the posterior spinal ligaments and fractures of the facet joints

Chapter 2

Clinical scales and scores

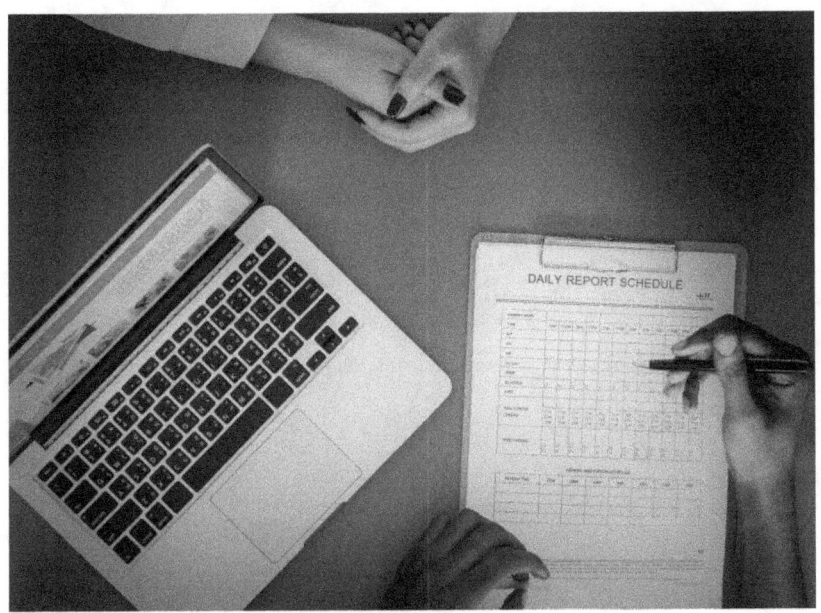

IN THIS CHAPTER

Neurology: Glasgow coma scale 57, National Institutes of Health Stroke Scale (NIHSS) 103.

Cardiopulmonary: CHA2DS2–VASc score 67, HAS-BLED score 69, Thrombolysis in myocardial infarction (TIMI) score 71, NYHA classification 94, GOLD criteria for COPD 95, Wells' score for pulmonary embolism 98, Revised Geneva Score for Pulmonary Embolism 99, Aortic Dissection Detection Risk Score (ADD-RS) 101.

Gastroenterology: Alvarado score 60, Forrest classification 63, Rockall score 64, Glasgow-Blatchford score 65, Child-Pugh score 72, West Haven Criteria 75, MELD score 77, Ranson Criteria 81, Glasgow prognostic score 83, classification of diverticular disease (CDD) 102.

Critical care: APACHE II Score 85, qSOFA criteria 89, Sequential Organ Failure Assessment (Sofa) score 90, Systemic Inflammatory Response Syndrome (SIRS) 97.

Anesthesiology: ASA Physical Status Classification System 88, VAS-Visual Analogue Scale 93, Mallampati score 96.

Miscellaneous: Karnofsky Performance Status scale 79, Performance Status Criteria 80.

Glasgow Coma Scale

Use

To estimate the level of consciousness

Scale[3]

Eye Opening (E)	Spontaneous	4
	To speech	3
	To pressure	2
	None	1
Verbal response (V)	Oriented	5
	Confused	4
	Words	3
	Sounds	2
	None	1
Best motor response (M)	Obeying commands	6
	Localizing	5
	Normal Flexion	4
	Abnormal Flexion	3
	Extension	2
	None	1

Always describe the individual components of the score as well as the sum. For example, GCS: 13, E4, V4, and M5.

Interpretion

The sum of the 3 categories is evaluated as follows
- 15   Normal consciousness level
- 14 to 4   Decreasing consciousness level
- 3   Deep coma

---

[3] www.glasgowcomascale.org

> **Warning**
> There is no GCS zero, even this book has a score of 3.
>
> If higher scores are encountered, please do not hesitate to ask for help! You already have a psychiatrist, right?

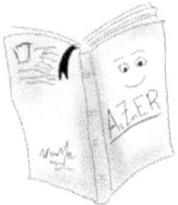

COMMENTS

- ✓ Response to pressure is elected by gentle pressure on finger tips.
- ✓ Oriented patient can correctly recognize time, place and persons.
- ✓ Response to pain is elected by Trapezius pinch or supraorbital pressure.
- ✓ Localization to pain means moving the hand above the clavicle in response to painful stimulus in head (supraorbital pressure) or neck (Trapezius pinch).
- ✓ Normal Flexion in response to painful stimulus: rapid flexion of the elbow joint with moving the hand away from the trunk.
- ✓ Abnormal flexion in response to painful stimulus: slow flexion of the elbow joint with moving the hand towards the trunk. Also the Forearm is pronated, the Thump is clenched and the lower limbs are extended.
- ✓ Extension in response to painful stimulus: extension of the elbow joint.
- ✓ Factors affecting the test result (False results):

Factors before the injury	Factors due to the injury
Dementia	Ocular trauma or orbital swelling
Hearing impairment	Drugs (anaesthetics, sedatives..etc)
Language barrier	Alcohol or drugs
	Limb or spinal-cord injuries

Clinical significance[4]

According to the NICE head injury guidelines

- GCS < 15 on initial assessment: Refer patients with head injury to a hospital.
- Suspected cervical spine injury:
    - GCS < 15 on initial assessment, apply a neck collar (cervical spine immobilization).
    - GCS<13 on initial assessment, order imaging of cervical spine (CT) within 1 hour.
- Indication of Brain CT (among others):
    - GCS < 13 on initial assessment.
    - GCS < 15 at 2 hours after the injury.
- Immediate intubation and ventilation GCS < 8

---

[4] According to the NICE head injury guidelines: www.nice.org.uk

Alvarado score

This scoring system is developed in 1986 by Dr. Alfredo Alvarado as a primary survey tool to help the clinical decision-making process regarding a suspected acute appendicitis.

Score[5]

	Criteria	Points
Symptoms	Migration/shifting of the pain	1
	Anorexia	1
	Nausea - Vomiting	1
Signs	Tenderness in right lower quadrant	2
	Rebound Tenderness (Blumberg sign)	1
	Elevated body temperature (>37.3°C measured orally)	1
Laboratory	Leukocytosis (>10 x10^9/L)	2
	Shift to the left (>75% neutrophils)	1

Comments

- ✓ MANTRELS mnemonic summarize the parameters of the score in the logical order of investigation; symptoms, signs and laboratory tests.
- ✓ The score is designed to be used for adult, non-pregnant patients with non-traumatic right iliac fossa pain. It can be misleading in extremities of age (younger as 10 years or older than 80 years). Also, false positive is more common with female patient due to the inability to exclude gynecological causes.
- ✓ Rovsing sign, the Dunphy's sign (cough test) or the Markle's test (heel-drop jarring test) can replace rebound tenderness.
- ✓ Headache is a very rare symptom in cases of acute appendicitis. When present subtract 2 points of the total score (Headache: -2 Points)

---

[5] Alvarado A. How to improve the clinical diagnosis of acute appendicitis in resource limited settings World Journal of Emergency Surgery. 2016; 11:16

- ✓ The score can be used as a method of evaluation and re-evaluation more than as a single tool for diagnosis. It is always advised to admit the patient with a reasonable clinical suspicion of appendicitis, then re-evaluate the situation every 4-6 hours, an increasing score here is more reliable for diagnosis than a single score value.
- ✓ The ideal situation is a young male patient with a score of 7 or more. Here you can proceed directly to surgical treatment with a reasonable confidence of your diagnosis.

INTERPRETATION

1-4	Appendicitis unlikely
5-6	Appendicitis possible
7-8	Appendicitis probable
9-10	Appendicitis very probable

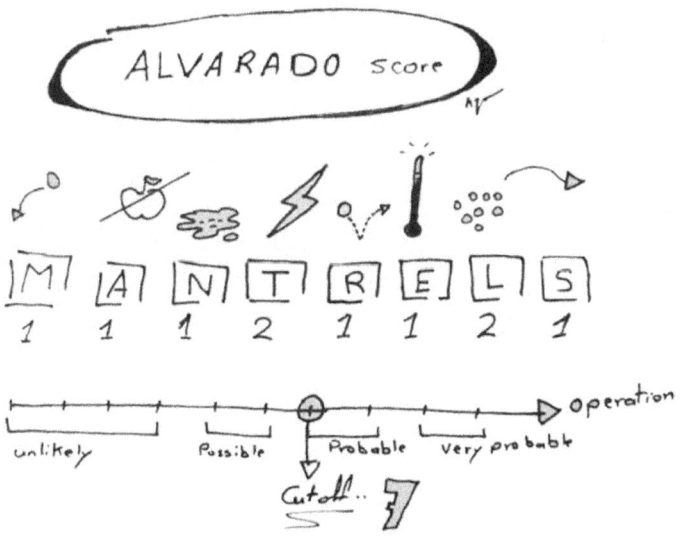

CLINICAL SIGNIFICANCE[6]

(Not applicable for trauma-related abdominal pain or pregnant patients)

It reasonable to use the clinical picture at first to determine the risk state of a patient with suspected acute appendicitis. According to the clinical picture further management decisions can be made. (Level B recommendations)

CT scan in adult patients with suspected acute appendicitis should be performed as abdominal and pelvic scan. Intravenous and oral contrast may increase the diagnostic value. (Level B recommendations)

Ultrasound in children can be used as a diagnostic tool to confirm the diagnosis but not to exclude it. It is a good specific positive tool with lower sensitivity. (Level B recommendations)

CT scan in children can be used to either confirm or exclude the diagnosis. It is a specific and sensitive test. (Level B recommendations)

In children, Ultrasound should be the first option in investigation. CT scan should be reserved of ambiguous or uncertain cases due to the risk of exposure to ionized radiations. (Level B recommendations)

---

[6] Howell JM, Eddy OL, Lukens TW, et al. Clinical Policy: critical issues in the evaluation and management of emergency department patients with suspected appendicitis. Ann Emerg Med. 2010;55:71-116.

Forrest classification

Use

Description of the endoscopic finding of upper GIT bleeding.

Classification

Acute hemorrhage	Forrest I a	Spurting hemorrhage
	Forrest I b	Oozing hemorrhage
Signs of recent hemorrhage	Forrest II a	Visible vessel
	Forrest II b	Adherent clot
	Forrest II c	Flat pigmented haematin on ulcer base
Lesions without active bleeding	Forrest III	Lesions without signs of recent hemorrhage or fibrin-covered clean ulcer base

Comments

✓ Forrest I and II stages are calculated in Rockall score as 2 points.

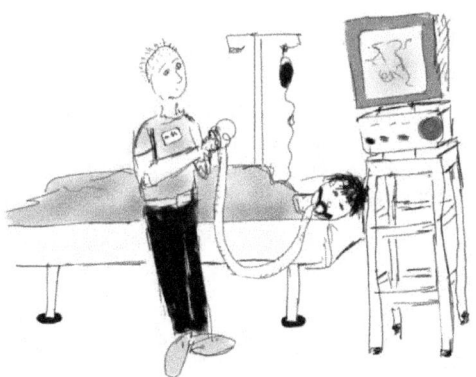

I am Forrest, Forrest Gump.
My Mama had always said
"the bleeding vessel always bleeds"

Rockall score

Use

Used for assessment of the risk of rebleeding in patient with upper gastrointestinal haemorrhage.

Score

	Score 0	Score 1	Score 2	Score 3
Age	<60	60-80	>80	
Shock	No	Pulse >100 Systolic BP >100	Systolic BP <100	
Co-morbidity			Congestive HF, Ischemic heart disease, other major morbidity	Renal failure, liver failure, metastatic cancer
Diagnosis/etiology	Mallory-Weiss Syndrome	All other diagnoses	GI malignancy	
Evidence of bleeding (endoscopic)			Blood, adherent clot or spurting vessel	

Interpretation

The sum of the points of the 5 factors determine the prognosis and rebleeding risk as follows:
- ➢ 0-2 Points: good prognosis, minor risk of rebleeding (5%)
- ➢ 3-8 Points: significant risk of rebleeding
- ➢ 8-11 Points: poor prognosis, significant risk of rebleeding and mortality.

Comments

- ✓ Rockall score can only be calculated after upper GIT endoscopy. It cannot be used as initial triage score.
- ✓ Mallory-Weiss Syndrome: Bleeding from a laceration a in the mucosa at the gastro-esophageal junction due to severe vomiting.
- ✓ Evidence of endoscopic bleeding is corresponding to Forrest classification I and II. *See Forrest classification.*

Glasgow-Blatchford score

Use

This is a screening tool to stratify patients with suspected upper GIT Bleeding according to the likelihood of the need of inpatient management.

Score

Criteria		Points
Hemoglobin (g/dL)	>13	0
	12-13	1
	10-12	3
	<10	6
BUN (mg/dL)	<18.2	0
	18.2-22.3	2
	22.4-28	3
	28-70	4
	>70	6
Systolic blood pressure (mm Hg)	≥110	0
	100–109	1
	90–99	2
	<90	3
Other criteria	Pulse ≥100 (per min)	1
	Melena present	1
	Presentation with syncope	2
	Liver disease history	2
	Heart failure history	2

Interpretation

The sum of all categories describes the risk class of the patient.
- ➢ 0 Points: very low risk, probability of intervention 0.5%
- ➢ 1-23 Points: increasing the risk of bleeding and the need of intervention.

COMMENTS

- ✓ The score is adjusted for women in Hemoglobin category as follows

>12	0
10-12	1
<10	6

- ✓ Score 0 patient profile:

  Male patient with Hb 13 g/dL or more (female with Hb 12 g/dL or more), BUN more than 18.2 mg/dL, systolic pressure more than 110 mm Hg and pulse frequency less than 100/min. The patient is presented with an attack of hematemesis without Melena. He/She gave no history of liver disease or heart failure.

CLINICAL SIGNIFICANCE

Both of the American College of Gastroenterology guidelines[7] and the British NICE guidelines of management of patients with upper GI Bleeding[8] indicated the importance of risk assessment of the patients as follows:

- Initial assessment using Glasgow-Blatchford score:
  - Score 0: discharge the patients with recommendation of outpatient upper GIT Endoscopy.
  - Score 1-23: Admission for inpatient management and stratify the patient for urgent endoscopy or ICU admission.
- After the Upper GIT endoscopy reassessment is carried out using Rockall score to judge further management steps including re-endoscopy, further monitoring or discharge timing.

---

[7] Management of Patients With Ulcer Bleeding. Am J Gastroenterol 2012; 107:345–360; doi: 10.1038/ajg.2011.480;

[8] Acute upper gastrointestinal bleeding in over 16s: management. nice.org.uk/guidance/cg141

CHA2DS2-VASc SCORE

USE

Evaluation of the long-term risk of stroke in atrial fibrillation (AF).

SCORE

C	Congestive Heart Failure	1
H	Hypertension	1
A2	Age > 75 years	2
D	Diabetes Mellitus	1
S2	Prior Stroke or TIA	2
V	Vascular disease	1
A	Age 65–74 years	1
Sc	Sex category (i.e. female sex)	1

INTERPRETATION

The sum of the 8 categories determines the annual risk of stroke in patients suffering from AF as follows:

- Score 0 (males) and 1 (females): low risk (0%)
- Score 1 (males) and 2 (females): moderate risk (1.3%)
- Score 2 -9 (males) and 3-9 (females): high risk (2.2% - 15.2%)

COMMENTS

- ✓ This is the updated version of the previously known CHADS2 score.
- ✓ The top score is 9 points not 10. Note that age category is doubled but its highest value is 2.
- ✓ Congestive Heart Failure: Signs/symptoms of heart failure or objective evidence of reduced left-ventricular ejection fraction
- ✓ Hypertension also includes cases well controlled under medication.
- ✓ DM: Fasting glucose >125 mg/dL (7 mmol/L) or treatment with oral hypoglycemic agent and/or insulin.
- ✓ Vascular disease includes: peripheral artery disease, myocardial infarction and aortic plaque.

CLINICAL SIGNIFICANCE

According to the European Society of Cardiology[9], the American College of Cardiology/American Heart Association[10] and NICE guidelines of AF management[11]

- The CHA2DS2-VASc score should be used to evaluate the risk of stroke in the following conditions:
    - Symptomatic or asymptomatic paroxysmal, persistent or permanent atrial fibrillation
    - Atrial flutter
    - A continuing risk of arrhythmia recurrence after cardioversion back to sinus rhythm.
- Anticoagulation prophylaxis should be considered according to CHA2DS2-VASc score as follows:
    - Score 0 (males) and 1 (females): no Anticoagulation prophylaxis.
    - Score 1 (males) and 2 (females): Anticoagulation prophylaxis is considered in patients with low risk of bleeding. See HAS-BLED score.
    - Score 2 -9 (males) and 3-9 (females): Anticoagulation prophylaxis is mandatory.

---

[9] 2016 ESC Guidelines for the management of atrial fibrillation developed in collaboration with EACTS. doi:10.1093/eurheartj/ehw210

[10] 2014 AHA/ACC/HRS Guideline for the Management of Patients with Atrial Fibrillation. http://www.onlinejacc.org/content/64/21/2246

[11] NICE guidelines, Atrial fibrillation: management – 2014, nice.org.uk/guidance/cg180

HAS-BLED SCORE

USE

Assessment of bleeding risk on oral anticoagulation in atrial fibrillation (AF)

SCORE

H	Hypertension: (uncontrolled, >160 mmHg systolic)	1
A	Abnormal renal function: Dialysis, transplant, Cr >2.26 mg/dL or >200 μmol/L	1
	Abnormal liver function: Cirrhosis or Bilirubin >2x Normal or AST/ALT/AP >3x Normal	1
S	Stroke: Prior history of stroke	1
B	Bleeding: Prior Major Bleeding or Predisposition to Bleeding	1
L	Labile INR: (Unstable/high INR), Time in therapeutic Range < 60%	1
E	Elderly: Age > 65 years	1
D	Drugs: Prior Alcohol or Drug Usage History (≥ 8 drinks/week)	1
	Drugs: Medication Usage Predisposing to Bleeding: (Antiplatelet agents, NSAIDs)	1

INTERPRETATION

The sum of all categories estimates the risk of major bleeding as follows:

- Score 0-1: low risk
- Score 2: moderate risk
- Score 3-9: high risk

CLINICAL SIGNIFICANCE

According to the European Society of Cardiology[12] and NICE guidelines of AF management[13]

- HAS-BLED score should be used to assess the risk of bleeding in patient receiving anticoagulation prophylaxis.
- Offer modification and monitoring of the following reversible risk factors:
    - Uncontrolled hypertension
    - Poor control of INR
    - Medication, for example concomitant use of aspirin or a non-steroidal
    - Anti-inflammatory drug (NSAID)
    - Excessive alcohol consumption.
- When discussing the benefits and risks of anticoagulation, explain to the person that:
    - For most people the benefit of anticoagulation outweighs the bleeding risk
    - For people with an increased risk of bleeding the benefit of anticoagulation may not always outweigh the bleeding risk, and careful monitoring of bleeding risk is important.
- Do not withhold anticoagulation solely because the person is at risk of having a fall.

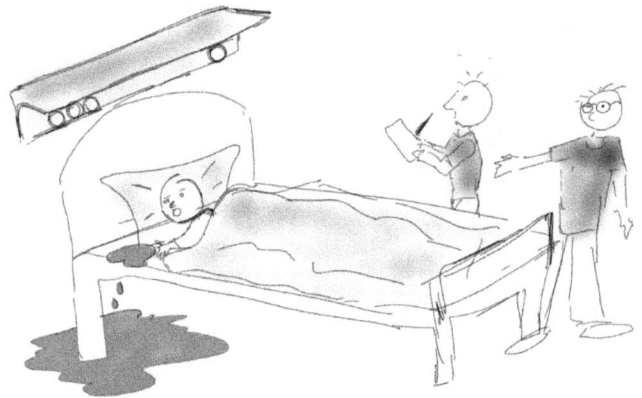

No need to calculate the score, the patient has already BLED!!

---

[12] 2016 ESC Guidelines for the management of atrial fibrillation developed in collaboration with EACTS. doi:10.1093/eurheartj/ehw210

[13] NICE guidelines, Atrial fibrillation: management – 2014, nice.org.uk/guidance/cg180

Thrombolysis in Myocardial Infarction (TIMI) Score

Use

TIMI score is used to determine the likelihood of ischemic events, urgent revascularization interventions or mortality in patients with unstable angina or non–ST-segment elevation myocardial infarction (NSTEMI) in the next 14 days.

Score

Age	≥65 years	1
Risk factors for coronary artery disease (CAD)	3 or more: family history of CAD, hypertension, hypercholesterolemia, diabetes mellitus, tobacco use	1
Known CAD	stenosis >50%	1
Aspirin	Aspirin use in the past 7 days	1
Severe angina	≥2 episodes in 24 hours	1
ECG	ST deviation ≥0.5 mm	1
Biomarker	Elevated cardiac marker level	1

Interpretation

The sum of all categories estimates the risk of ischemic events, urgent revascularization interventions or mortality as follows:

Score	Risk
0-1	5%
2	8%
3	13%
4	20%
5	26%
6-7	41%

```
Mnemonic ABCDE:

A Age, Aspirin, Angina
B Biomarker
C CAD risk factors
D Diagnosis of CAD
E ECG changes
```

Child-Pugh score

Use

To determine the severity of liver functions impairment.

Scale[14]

Factors	Points		
	1	2	3
Total bilirubin (µmol/L)	<34	34-50	>50
Serum albumin (g/L)	>35	35-28	<28
INR	<1.7	1.7-2.3	>2.30
Ascites	None	Mild	Moderate to severe
Hepatic encephalopathy	None	Grade I-II (or suppressed with medication)	Grade III-IV (or refractory)

Interpretation

The sum of the points of the 5 factors determine the class as follows:

- Class A: 5 – 6 Points
- Class B: 7 – 9 Points
- Class C: 10 – 15 Points

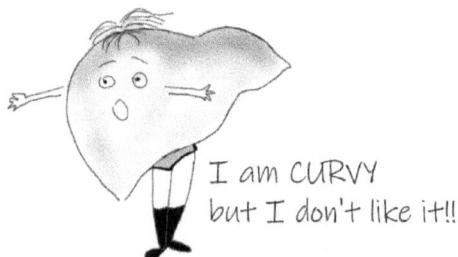

I am CURVY but I don't like it!!

---

[14] Walker HK, Hall WD, Hurst JW. Clinical Methods: The History, Physical, and Laboratory Examinations. 3rd edition. Boston: Butterworths; 1990.

COMMENTS

- ✓ Synonym: The Child-Turcott-Pugh (CTP) score.
- ✓ Alternative units of measuring total bilirubin is mg/dL and for serum albumin is g/dL. Accordingly the points are assigned as follows:

	1	2	3
Total bilirubin (mg/dL)	<2	2-3	>3
Serum albumin (g/dL)	>3.5	3.5-2.8	<2.8

- ✓ Mild ascites (less than 500 ml) is not detected clinically. It can only be detected using imaging techniques as CT or Ultrasound. On the other hand the clinically detected ascites is considered moderate (shifting dullness sign) to severe (fluid thrill wave sign).
- ✓ Hepatic encephalopathy Grade (see West Haven Criteria)

CLINICAL SIGNIFICANCE[15]

- Determine the correlation between liver cirrhosis and liver functions
    - Class A: well compensated liver functions. Good liver physiological reserve.
    - Class B: significant functional deterioration, borderline physiological liver reserve
    - Class C: decompensated liver function. Depleted liver physiological reserve.
- Asses 1-year life expectancy
    - Class A: 100%
    - Class B: 80%
    - Class C: 45%
- Asses 2-year life expectancy
    - Class A: 85%
    - Class B: 60%
    - Class C: 35%
- Asses perioperative mortality In cirrhotic patients who undergo abdominal surgery
    - Class A: 10%
    - Class B: 30–31%
    - Class C: 76–82%
- Decision making regarding the management of hepatocellular carcinoma (among other criteria)
    - Class A: surgical resection could be considered

---

[15] A James Hanje; Tushar Patel, Preoperative Evaluation of Patients with Liver Disease, Nat Clin Pract Gastroenterol Hepatol. 2007;4(5):266-276.

- - Class B: less invasive palliative options are indicated (e.g. Radiofrequency ablation RFA or transcatheter arterial chemoembolization-TACE)
  - Class C: mostly supportive treatment
- Child-Pugh score is integrated in other scoring systems. For example the Cancer of Liver Italian Program (CLIP) prognostic system for hepatocellular carcinoma.

WEST HAVEN CRITERIA

USE

Grading of hepatic encephalopathy or the mental state deterioration accompanying liver cell failure.

SCALE[16]

Grade I	Trivial lack of awareness
	Sleep disorder
	Shortened attention span
	Euphoria or depression
	Asterixis or tremor
Grade II	Lethargy
	Disorientation to time
	Amnesia of recent events
	Inappropriate behavior
	Anxiety
	Slurred speech
	Hyperactive reflexes
Grade III	Somnolence (sleepiness) to stupor
	Confusion
	Gross disorientation
	Bizarre behavior
	Babinski reflex,
	rigidity
Grade IV	Coma (unresponsive to verbal/painful stimuli) - GCS 3

---

[16] Ferenci P, Lockwood A, Mullen K, Tarter R, Weissenborn K, Blei AT. Hepatic encephalopathy—definition, nomenclature, diagnosis, and quantification: final report of the working party at the 11th World Congresses of Gastroenterology, Vienna, 1998. Hepatology. 2002;35:716-21.

Comments

- ✓ Asterixis: flapping tremors of the extended hands.
- ✓ Stupor is the lack of critical cognitive functions and the level of consciousness. The patient only responds to base stimuli such as pain.
- ✓ The Babinski reflex occurs when the sole of the foot has been firmly stroked. Negative reflex (normal) is the plantar flexion of all toes. Positive Babinski reflex is the dorsiflexion of the big toe and the fanning of the other toes. It is a normal reflex only in infants.

MELD SCORE

USE

Model of End Stage Liver Disease

SCORE[17]

Candidates who are at least 12 years old receive an initial MELD(i) score equal to:

MELD(i) = 0.957 × ln(Cr) + 0.378 × ln(bilirubin) + 1.120 × ln(INR) + 0.643

Then, round to the tenth decimal place and multiply by 10. Maximum MELD = 40.

If MELD(i) > 11, perform additional MELD calculation as follows:

MELD = MELD(i) + 1.32 × (137 − Na) − [0.033 × MELD(i) × (137 − Na)]

COMMENTS

The MELD score calculation uses:
- Serum Creatinine (mg/dl)
- Bilirubin (mg/dl)
- INR
- Serum Sodium (mEq/L)

ONLINE CALCULATOR

Provided by the Organ Procurement and Transplantation Network (OPTN) - U.S. Department of Health & Human Services

---

[17] Cirrhosis in over 16s: assessment and management NICE guideline. Published: 6 July 2016. *nice.org.uk/guidance/ng50*

LINK

https://optn.transplant.hrsa.gov/resources/allocation-calculators/meld-calculator/

CLINICAL SIGNIFICANCE

- Monitoring of patients suffering from liver cirrhosis. (NICE guideline)
    - Calculate the MELD score every 6 months for people with compensated cirrhosis (Child-A Patients).
    - A MELD score of 12 or more is an indicator an impending risk of complications of cirrhosis.
- Organ Procurement and Transplantation Network (OPTN) Policies – USA
    - MELD score is used to stratify candidates of liver transplantation waiting list according to the probabilities of death within a 3-month period.

Karnofsky Performance Status Scale

Use

Scale used to evaluate the effect of the malignant disease on the general health status of the patient.

Scale[18]

100%	Normal no complaints; no evidence of disease.
90%	Able to carry on normal activity; minor signs or symptoms of disease.
80%	Normal activity with effort; some signs or symptoms of disease.
70%	Cares for self; unable to carry on normal activity or to do active work.
60%	Requires occasional assistance, but is able to care for most of his personal needs.
50%	Requires considerable assistance and frequent medical care.
40%	Disabled; requires special care and assistance.
30%	Severely disabled; hospital admission is indicated although death not imminent.
20%	Very sick; hospital admission necessary; active supportive treatment necessary.
10%	Moribund; fatal processes progressing rapidly.
0%	Dead

Interpretation

➢ **100% - 80%:** The patient is able to carry on normal activity and to work; no special care needed.
➢ **70% - 50%:** The patient is unable to work; able to live at home and care for most personal needs; varying amount of assistance are needed.
➢ **40% or below:** The patient is unable to care for self; requires equivalent of institutional or hospital care; disease may be progressing rapidly.

---

[18] Crooks, V, Waller S, et al. The use of the Karnofsky Performance Scale in determining outcomes and risk in geriatric outpatients. J Gerontol. 1991; 46: M139-M144

Performance Status Criteria

Use

Eastern Cooperative Oncology Group (ECOG) Performance Status Criteria is used to evaluate the effect of the malignant disease on the general health status of the patient.

Scale[19]

0	Fully active, able to carry on all pre-disease performance without restriction
1	Restricted in physically strenuous activity but ambulatory and able to carry out work of a light or sedentary nature, e.g., light house work, office work
2	Ambulatory and capable of all selfcare but unable to carry out any work activities. Up and about more than 50% of waking hours
3	Capable of only limited selfcare, confined to bed or chair more than 50% of waking hours
4	Completely disabled. Cannot carry on any selfcare. Totally confined to bed or chair
5	Dead

Comments

This scale is equivalent to the Karnofsky Performance status scale.

Performance Status scale	Karnofsky scale
0	100% – 90%
1	80% -70%
2	60% - 50%
3	40% -30%
4	20% - 10%
5	0%

---

[19] Oken, M.M., Creech, R.H., Tormey, D.C., Horton, J., Davis, T.E., McFadden, E.T., Carbone, P.P.: Toxicity And Response Criteria Of The Eastern Cooperative Oncology Group. Am J Clin Oncol 5:649-655, 1982.

RANSON CRITERIA

USE

Used for determining the prognosis (mortality) and severity in patients with acute pancreatitis.

CRITERIA FOR NON-GALLSTONE PANCREATITIS

Calculated on admission		Calculated after 48 hours	
Age	>55 years	Haematocrit fall	>10%
Serum glucose	200 mg/dL (11.1 mmols/L)	Estimated fluid sequestration	>6 L
WBC count	>16 x 10^3/microlitre (16 x10^9/L)	Base deficit	>4 mEq/L
Serum AST (SGOT)	>250 units/L	BUN rise	>5 mg/dL (1.8 mmols/L)
Serum LDH	>350 units/L	Serum Calcium	<8 mg/dL (2 mmols/L)
		Arterial PO2 on room air	<60 mmHg (8 kPa)

CRITERIA FOR GALLSTONE PANCREATITIS

Calculated on admission		Calculated after 48 hours	
Age	>70 years	Haematocrit fall	>10%
Serum glucose	220 mg/dL (12.2 mmols/L)	Estimated fluid sequestration	>4 L
WBC count	>18 x 10^3/microlitre (18 x10^9/L)	Base deficit	>5 mEq/L
Serum AST (SGOT)	>250 units/L	BUN rise	>2 mg/dL (0.7 mmols/L)
Serum LDH	>400 units/L	Serum Calcium	<8 mg/dL (2 mmols/L)

INTERPRETATION

1 point is assigned for each positive criterion. The sum of the points predicts the mortality probability as follows:

- 0 - 2 = 0%
- 3 - 4 = 15%
- 5 - 6 = 50%
- \>6 = 100%

COMMENTS

- ✓ The Ranson score can only be calculated after 48 hours after diagnosis (admission).
- ✓ Initial (on admission) Hematocrit and Blood Urea Nitrogen (BUN) values must be available to calculate the Ranson score.
- ✓ In case of incomplete data (for example due to missing laboratory value) the score can also be calculated using the available values but the score now represents the least possible value. For example the score without BUN initial value will be at least 3 points, so the mortality probability is at least 15%.

Glasgow prognostic score

Use

Used for determining the severity in patients with acute pancreatitis.

Criteria

Age	>55 years
Serum albumin	<3.2 g/dL (32 g/L)
Arterial PO2 on room air	<60 mmHg (8 kPa)
Serum calcium	<8 mg/dL (2 mmols/L)
Serum Blood urea nitrogen	>16.1 mg/dL (45 mmols/L)
Serum LDH	>600 units/L
Serum glucose	180 mg/dL (10 mmols/L)
WBC count	>15 x 10^3/microlitre (15 x10^9/L)

Interpretation

1 point is assigned for each positive criterion. Severe acute pancreatitis is predicted when the sum is 3 or more.

Comments

- ✓ Synonym: Imrie's criteria
- ✓ The score can be calculated any time in the first 48 hours

CLINICAL SIGNIFICANCE

- According to UK guidelines for the management of acute pancreatitis[20], Glasgow prognostic score could be used to determine severe acute pancreatitis.
- According to the official recommendations of the American Gastroenterological Association (AGA) Institute on "Management of Acute Pancreatitis[21]
    - A severe acute pancreatitis is determined using APACHI II score equal to or more than 8.
    - Intensive care unit admission is mandatory in patients with confirmed or predicted severe pancreatitis.
    - Abdominal CT scan – *if not otherwise indicated* – should be first carried out after 72 hours to detect necrotizing pancreatitis.
    - Laboratory tests can be used as an adjunct to clinical judgment and the APACHE II score. For example: serum C-reactive protein level of >150 mg/L at 48 indicates a severe course.

---

[20] UK guidelines for the management of acute pancreatitis. http://dx.doi.org/10.1136/gut.2004.057026

[21] The recommendations of the American Gastroenterological Association (AGA) Institute on "Management of Acute Pancreatitis. http://www.gastro.org/guidelines/acute-pancreatitis#sec1.2

APACHE II Score

Use

Acute Physiology and Chronic Health Evaluation. Estimates the mortality of adult patients admitted to intensive care units.

Score[22]

	4	3	2	1	0	1	2	3	4
Temperature, core (°C)	≥41°	39–40.9°		38.5–38.9°	36–38.4°	34–35.9°	32–33.9°	30–31.9°	≤29.9°
Mean arterial pressure (mm Hg)	≥160	130–159	110–129	—	70–109	—	50–69	—	≤49
Heart rate	≥180	140–179	110–139	—	70–109	—	55–69	40–54	≤39
Respiratory rate (nonventilated or ventilated)	≥50	35–49	—	25–34	12–24	10–11	6–9	—	≤5
Oxygenation[23]: A-aDO$_2$	≥500	350–499	200–349	—	< 200	—	—	—	—
P$_{AO_2}$ (mm Hg)	—	—	—	—	> 70	61–70	—	55–60	< 55
Arterial pH	≥7.7	7.6–7.69	—	7.5–7.59	7.33–7.49	—	7.25–7.32	7.15–7.24	< 7.15

---

[22] https://reference.medscape.com/calculator/apache-ii-scoring-system
[23] Oxygenation: a) FIO2≥0.5: use A-aDO2 OR b) FIO_2<0.5: use PAO_2 (mm Hg)

Serum Na (mmol/L)	≥ 180	160–179	155–159	150–154	**130–149**	—	120–129	111–119	≤ 110
Serum K (mmol/L)	≥ 7	6–6.9	—	5.5–5.9	**3.5–5.4**	3–3.4	2.5–2.9	—	< 2.5
Serum creatinine (mg/dL)[24]	≥ 3.5	2–3.4	1.5–1.9	—	**0.6–1.4**	—	< 0.6	—	—
Hct (%)	≥ 60	—	50–59.9	46–49.9	**30–45.9**	—	20–29.9	—	< 20
WBC (in 1000s)	≥ 40	—	20–39.9	15–19.9	**3–14.9**	—	1–2.9	—	< 1
Glasgow coma score (GCS)				Score = 15 minus actual GCS					
Age				Add 0 points for age <44; 2 points, 45–54 yr; 3 points, 55–64 yr; 5 points, 65–74 yr; 6 points ≥ 75 yr.					
Chronic health status				2 points for elective postoperative patient with immunocompromise or history of severe organ insufficiency; 5 points for nonoperative patient or emergency postoperative patient with immunocompromise or severe organ insufficiency (hepatic, cardiovascular, renal or pulmonary)					

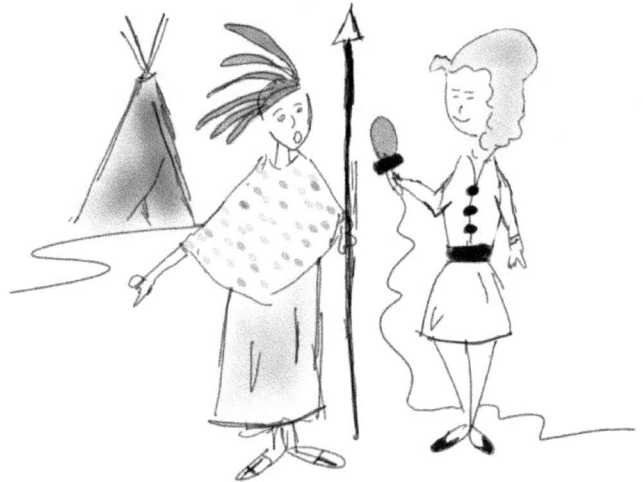

No!! We have nothing to do with the ICU mortality!!

---

[24] double point score for **acute renal failure**

COMMENTS

- ✓ Many online calculators are available. For example, check out this link: https://reference.medscape.com/calculator/apache-ii-scoring-system

- ✓ Choose worst value on admission or in the past 24 h.

- ✓ Chronic Health Problems: 1) Cirrhosis of the liver confirmed by biopsy 2) New York Heart Association Class IV 3) Severe COPD -- Hypercapnia, home O2 use, or pulmonary hypertension 4) On regular dialysis or 5) Immunocompromised

INTERPRETATION

The sum of the first 12 criteria represents the acute physiological score. By adding the age and the chronic health status score we obtain the Acute Physiology and Chronic Health Evaluation score, AKA APACHE II Score.

APACHE II SCORE	Hospital mortality (%)	
	Non-operative	Postoperative
0-4	4	1
5-9	6	3
10-14	12	6
15-19	22	11
20-24	40	29
24-29	51	37
30-34	71	71
More than 34	82	87

ASA PHYSICAL STATUS CLASSIFICATION SYSTEM

Use

Assessing the fitness of patients before surgery. Developed by the American Society of Anesthesiologists.

Scale[25]

ASA I	A normal healthy patient
ASA II	A patient with mild systemic disease
ASA III	A patient with severe systemic disease
ASA IV	A patient with severe systemic disease that is a constant threat to life
ASA V	A moribund patient who is not expected to survive without the operation
ASA VI	A declared brain-dead patient whose organs are being removed for donor purposes

---

[25] https://www.asahq.org/resources/clinical-information/asa-physical-status-classification-system

QSOFA CRITERIA

USE

Identify patients with suspected sepsis who should have further clinical and laboratory investigation.

CRITERIA[26]

- Respiratory rate ≥ 22/min
- Altered mentation
- Systolic BP ≤ 100 mm Hg

(at least 2 criteria must be present)

> When a patient with known infection sets on the SOFA (Panting, feeling light-headed and acting weird), it is always a bad sign. Septic shock impending.

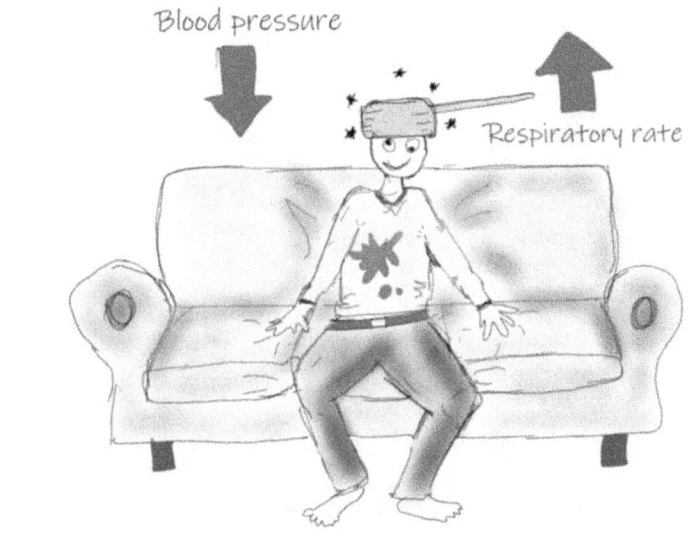

---

[26] Singer M, Deutschman CS, Seymour CW, et al. The Third International Consensus Definitions for Sepsis and Septic Shock (Sepsis-3). JAMA. 2016;315(8):801–810. doi:10.1001/jama.2016.0287

Sequential Organ Failure Assessment (SOFA) Score

Use

Prognosis, mortality and prediction of multiple organ failure in patient with sepsis in the intensive care unit.

Score

	0	1	2	3	4
Pao_2/FIO_2	≥ 400 mm Hg (53.3 kPa)	< 400 mm Hg (53.3 kPa)	< 300 mm Hg (40 kPa)	< 200 mm Hg (26.7 kPa) with respiratory support	< 100 mm Hg (13.3 kPa) with respiratory support
Platelets × $10^3/\mu L$	≥ 150	< 150	< 100	< 50	< 20
Bilirubin	≥ 1.2 mg/dL (20 µmol/L)	1.2–1.9 mg/dL (20–32 µmol/L)	2.0–5.9 mg/dL (33–101 µmol/L)	6.0–11.9 mg/dL (102–204 µmol/L)	> 12.0 mg/dL (204 µmol/L)
Cardiovascular	MAP ≥ 70 mm Hg	MAP < 70 mm Hg	Dopamine < 5 mcg/kg/min for ≥ 1 h or Any dose of dobutamine	Dopamine 5.1–15 mcg/kg/min for ≥ 1 h or Epinephrine ≤ 0.1 mcg/kg/min for ≥ 1 h or Norepinephrine ≤ 0.1 mcg/kg/min for ≥ 1 h	Dopamine > 15 mcg/kg/min for ≥ 1 h or Epinephrine > 0.1 mcg/kg/min for ≥ 1 h or Norepinephrine > 0.1 mcg/kg/min for ≥ 1 h
Glasgow coma score (GCS)	15 points	13–14 points	10–12 points	6–9 points	< 6 points
Creatinine	< 1.2 mg/dL (110 µmol/L)	1.2-1.9 mg/dL (110–170 µmol/L)	2.0-3.4 mg/dL (171–299 µmol/L)	3.5-4.9 mg/dL (300–400 µmol/L)	> 5.0 mg/dL (440 µmol/L)
Urine output	—	—	—	< 500 mL/day	< 200 mL/day

FIO2 = fractional inspired O2; kPa = kilopascals; MAP = mean arterial pressure; Pao2 = arterial oxygen partial pressure.

COMMENTS

- ✓ The baseline SOFA score can be assumed to be zero in patients not known to have preexisting organ dysfunction.
- ✓ The score covers various body systems to detect multiple organ failure.

INTERPRETATION

SOFA score ≥2 points = Organ dysfunction consequent to the infection (Sepsis-related organ failure).

SOFA score ≥2 points = mortality risk of approximately 10% in a general hospital population with suspected infection.

CLINICAL SIGNIFICANCE

As proposed by The Third International Consensus Definitions for Sepsis and Septic Shock (Sepsis-3)[27]

---

[27] Singer M, Deutschman CS, Seymour CW, et al. The Third International Consensus Definitions for Sepsis and Septic Shock (Sepsis-3). JAMA. 2016;315(8):801–810. doi:10.1001/jama.2016.0287

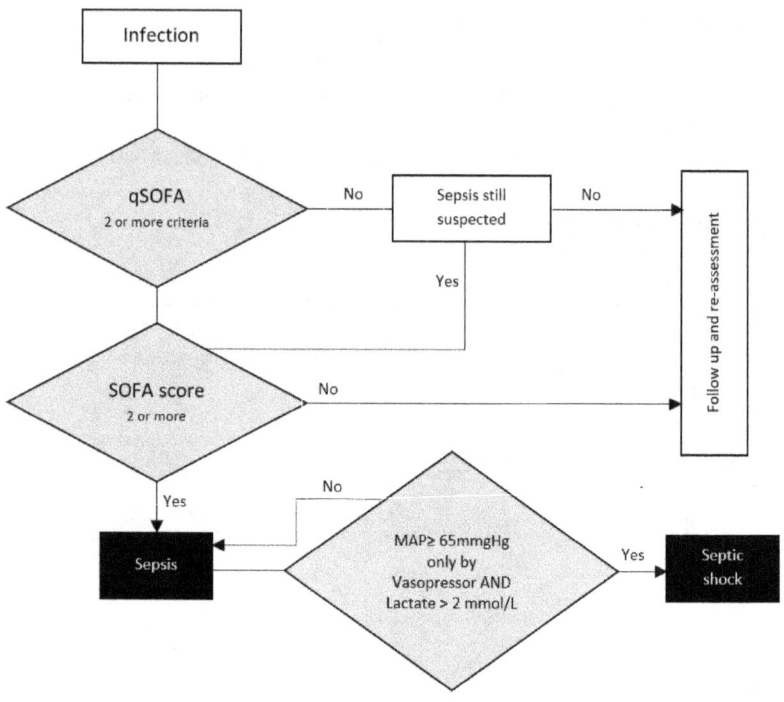

VAS-Visual Analogue Scale

Use

Subjective assessment of pain severity.

Scale

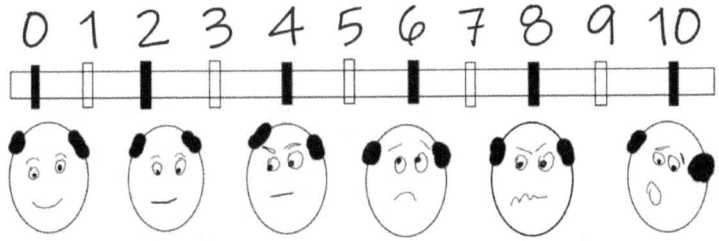

Interpretation

0	no pain
2	Mild pain
4	Moderate pain
6	Severe pain
8	Very severe pain
10	Excruciating pain

Comments

This a subjective score. The patient describes his pain in terms of numbers where zero is no pain at all and 10 is the worst possible pain ever. It is obvious that a lot of personal factors can affect the outcome of this score. This why this score could never be used to compare the pain severity in 2 different patients. But on the other hand, it is most useful in the follow up of the pain severity of the same patient. Also, it is widely used in triage systems of ER.

NYHA Classification

Use

New York Heart Association (NYHA) Functional Classification of the severity of heart failure.

Scale[28]

Class	Patient Symptoms
I	No limitation of physical activity. *Ordinary physical activity does not cause undue fatigue, palpitation, dyspnea.*
II	Slight limitation of physical activity. *Comfortable at rest. Ordinary physical activity results in fatigue, palpitation, dyspnea.*
III	Marked limitation of physical activity. *Comfortable at rest. Less than ordinary activity causes fatigue, palpitation, or dyspnea.*
IV	Unable to carry on any physical activity without discomfort. *Symptoms of heart failure at rest. If any physical activity is undertaken, discomfort increases.*
Class	Objective Assessment
A	No objective evidence of cardiovascular disease. No symptoms and no limitation in ordinary physical activity.
B	Objective evidence of minimal cardiovascular disease. Mild symptoms and slight limitation during ordinary activity. Comfortable at rest.
C	Objective evidence of moderately severe cardiovascular disease. Marked limitation in activity due to symptoms, even during less-than-ordinary activity. Comfortable only at rest.
D	Objective evidence of severe cardiovascular disease. Severe limitations. Experiences symptoms even while at rest.

Each patient is assigned 2 classes: Function Capacity class (I to IV) and Objective Assessment class (A to D).

---

[28] https://www.heart.org/en/health-topics/heart-failure/what-is-heart-failure/classes-of-heart-failure

GOLD Criteria for COPD

Use

Global Initiative for Obstructive Lung Disease (GOLD) Criteria for the classification of airflow limitation severity in COPD.

Scale[29]

		The forced expiratory volume in one second (FEV1)
GOLD 1	Mild airflow limitation	FEV1 ≥ 80% predicted
GOLD 2	Moderate airflow limitation	50% ≤ FEV1 < 80% predicted
GOLD 3	Severe airflow limitation	30% ≤ FEV1 < 50% predicted
GOLD 4	Very severe airflow limitation	FEV1 < 30% predicted

Comments

- ✓ Specific spirometric cut-points are used for purposes of simplicity.
- ✓ Spirometry should be performed after the administration of an adequate dose of at least one short-acting inhaled bronchodilator in order to minimize variability.

---

[29] Pocket guide to copd diagnosis, management, and prevention of COPD – 2017, https://goldcopd.org/gold-reports-2017/

Mallampati score

Use

It describes the relationship between tongue and oropharynx, when the patient maximally opens his mouth, protrudes his tongue and say AAA (to elevate the soft palate maximally).

Scale

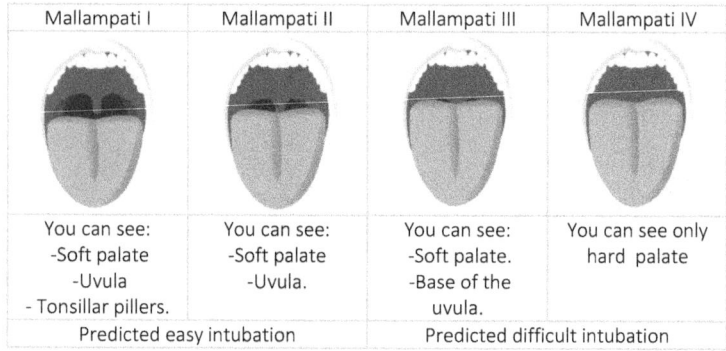

Mallampati I	Mallampati II	Mallampati III	Mallampati IV
You can see: -Soft palate -Uvula - Tonsillar pillers.	You can see: -Soft palate -Uvula.	You can see: -Soft palate. -Base of the uvula.	You can see only hard palate
Predicted easy intubation		Predicted difficult intubation	

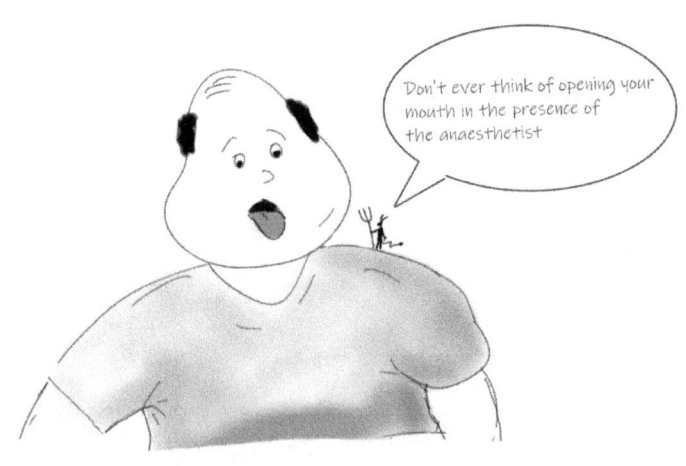

Don't ever think of opening your mouth in the presence of the anaesthetist

Systemic Inflammatory Response Syndrome (SIRS)

Use

This a generalized response to trauma characterized by release of inflammatory mediators. It is associated with conditions such as, disseminated intravascular coagulopathy (DIC), acute respiratory distress syndrome (ARDS), renal failure, multisystem organ failure (MOF) and shock.

Score

Variable	Value	Points
Heart rate	> 90 beats/min	1
WBC count	<4000cells/mm^3 OR >12,000 cells/mm^3	1
Respiratory rate	rate > 20	1
Temperature	< 36 degrees OR > 38 degrees	1

Interpretation

score of 2 or more meets criteria for SIRS

Wells' Score for Pulmonary Embolism

Use

Estimate the risk of pulmonary embolism (PE).

Score

Criteria	Points
Clinical signs and symptoms of deep venous thrombosis (DVT)	3
PE is the most likely diagnosis OR equally likely to other differential diagnosis	3
Heart rate > 100 b.p.m.	1.5
Immobilization at least 3 days OR surgery in the previous 4 weeks	1.5
Past history of PE or DVT	1.5
Hemoptysis	1
Malignancy treatment within 6 months (curative or palliative)	1

Interpretation

Three level score of clinical probability	
Low probability of PE	0-1
Intermediate probability of PE	2-6
High probability of PE	7 or more
Two level score of clinical probability	
unlikely	0-4
likely	5 or more

Comments

One of the disadvantages of this score is the second criterion which can be considered subjective. The estimate of the PE as the most likely diagnosis depends mainly on the user experience and leave a wide space of variation in test results carried out by different users[30].

---

[30] Gruettner J, Walter T, Lang S, Meyer M, Apfaltrer P, Henzler T, Viergutz T, Importance of Wells score and Geneva score for the evaluation of patients suspected of pulmonary embolism. In Vivo. 2015 Mar-Apr;29(2):269-72.

Revised Geneva Score for Pulmonary Embolism

Use

Estimate the risk of pulmonary embolism (PE).

Score

Criteria	Points
Tenderness in calf muscles or unilateral lower limb oedema	4
Unilateral lower limb pain	3
Heart rate 75-94 b.p.m.	3
Heart rate >94 b.p.m.	5
Fracure OR surgery in the previous 4 weeks	2
Past history of PE or DVT	3
Hemoptysis	2
Active Malignancy (treatment in the past 12 months)	2
Age >65 years	1

Interpretation

Three level score of clinical probability
Low probability of PE   0-3
Intermediate probability of PE 4-10
High probability of PE   11 or more
Two level score of clinical probability
unlikely   0-5
likely   6 or more

Comments

While CT Angiography remains the gold standard for the diagnosis of PE, both Wells' Score and the revised Geneva score are handy tools in the initial management of Hemodynamically stable patients.

The European Society of Cardiology suggests the use of either of the two scores to guide the clinical decision making. Also, for the interpretation you are free to the three-level score (low, intermediate or high probability of PE) or the two-level score (PE likely or PE unlikely).

Aortic Dissection Detection Risk Score (ADD-RS)

Use

Diagnosis of possible aortic dissection.

Score

Category	High risk factors	Points (maximum 1 point for each category)
History	Marfan syndrome Positive family history of aortic disease Aortic valve disease Known thoracic aortic aneurysm Previous aortic interventions or operations	1
Symptoms	Thoracic, back or abdominal pain with at least one of the following abrupt onset Severe pain Tearing pain	1
Investigation	Evidence of perfusion deficit such as Pulse deficit Systolic blood pressure differential (bilateral or upper/lower limb) Focal neurological deficit with pain Hypotension or shock New aortic insufficiency murmur	1

Interpretation

- ✓ 0 or 1: procced to D-Dimer.
    - o Negative D-Dimer: Aortic dissection is unlikely, look for the differential diagnosis.
    - o Positive D-Dimer: Aortic dissection is likely. Proceed to CT.
- ✓ More than 1: Aortic dissection is likely. Proceed directly to CT.

Classification of Diverticular Disease (CDD)

Use

A recent clinically oriented scale for the classification of diverticular disease.

Scale

Type	Subtype
Type 0: asymptomatic diverticulosis	
Type 1: acute uncomplicated diverticulitis	1a: without peridiverticulitis 1b: with peridiverticulitis
Type 2: acute complicated diverticulitis	All are diverticulitis with peridiverticulitis with one of the following complications: 2a: microabscesses (less than 1 cm size abscesses or concealed perforation) 2b: with macroabscesses (more than 1 cm size paracolic or mesocolic abscesses) 2c: free perforation 2c1: with purulent peritonitis 2c2: with fecal peritonitis
Type 3: chronic diverticulitis	3a: symptomatic uncomplicated diverticular disease 3b: relapsing uncomplicated diverticular disease 3c: relapsing complicated diverticular disease (stenosis, fistula or conglomerate tumor)
Type 4: diverticular bleeding	

NATIONAL INSTITUTES OF HEALTH STROKE SCALE (NIHSS)

USE

Determine the severity of a cerebrovascular stroke.

SCALE

Level of Consciousness (Responsiveness)		
score	How to perform: Observation of the patient	Measures the initial level of consciousness
0	Alert; Responsive	
1	Not alert; Verbally arousable or aroused by minor stimulation to obey, answer, or respond.	
2	Not alert; Only responsive to repeated or strong and painful stimuli	
3	Totally unresponsive; Responds only with reflexes or is areflexic	
Notes: if the patient score in this category is 3, the default coma score should be assigned in the next categories when applicable		
Level of Consciousness (Questions)		
score	How to perform: Patient is verbally asked his or her age and for the name of the current month.	Left cortical function
0	Correctly answers both questions	
1	Correctly answers one question	
2	Does not correctly answer either question	
Notes ✓ Default Coma Score: 2 ✓ The patient must answer each question 100% correct without help to get credit ✓ Patients unable to speak are allowed to write the answer ✓ Aphasic patients or patients in a stuporous state who are unable to understand the commands receive a score of 2 ✓ Patients that are unable to talk due to trauma, dysarthria, language barrier, or intubation are given a score of 1		
Level of Consciousness (Commands)		

score	How to perform: The patient is instructed to first open and close his or her eyes and then grip and release his or her hand
0	Correctly performs both tasks
1	Correctly performs 1 task
2	Does not correctly perform either task
Notes	✓ Commands can only be repeated once. ✓ The hand grip command can be replaced with any other simple one step command if the patient cannot use his or her hands. ✓ A patient's attempt is regarded as successful if an attempt is made but is incomplete due to weakness

Horizontal Eye Movement

score	How to perform: Assesses ability for patient to track a pen or finger from side to side only using his or her eyes.
0	Normal; Able to follow pen or finger to both sides
1	Partial gaze palsy; gaze is abnormal in one or both eyes, but gaze is not totally paralyzed. Patient can gaze towards hemisphere of infarct, but can't go past midline
2	Total gaze paresis; gaze is fixed to one side
Notes	✓ If patient is unable to follow the command to track an object, the investigator can make eye contact with the patient and then move side to side. The patient's gaze palsy can then be assessed by his or her ability to maintain eye contact.

Visual field test

score	How to perform: Assess the patient's vision in each visual fields. Each eye is tested individually, by covering one eye and then the other. Each upper and lower quadrant is tested by asking the patient to indicate how many fingers the investigator is presenting in each quadrant. The investigator should instruct the patient to maintain eye contact throughout this test, and not allow the patient to realign focus towards each stimulus.
0	No vision loss
1	Partial hemianopia or complete quadrantanopia; patient recognizes no visual stimulus in one specific quadrant
2	Complete hemianopia; patient recognizes no visual stimulus in one half of the visual field
3	Bilateral Blindness, including blindness from any cause
Notes	✓ If patient is not responsive the visual fields can be tested by visual threat (the investigator moving an object towards the eye and

Left cortical function

observing the patient's response, being careful not to trigger the corneal reflex with air movement).

Facial Palsy

score	How to perform: While inspecting the symmetry of each facial expression the examiner should first instruct patient to show his or her teeth. Second, the patient should be asked to squeeze his or her eyes closed as hard as possible. After reopening his or her eyes, the patient is then instructed to raise his or her eyebrows.
0	Normal and symmetrical movement
1	Minor paralysis; function is less than clearly normal, such as flattened nasolabial fold or minor asymmetry in smile
2	Partial paralysis; particularly paralysis in lower face
3	Complete facial Hemiparesis, total paralysis in upper and lower portions of one face side

Notes
- ✓ Patients incapable of comprehending an commands may be tested by applying a noxious stimulus and observing for any paralysis in the resulting grimace.

Motor Arm

score	How to perform: With palm facing downwards, have the patient extend one arm 90 degrees out in front if the patient is sitting, and 45 degrees out in front if the patient is lying down. If necessary, help the patient get into the correct position. As soon as the patient's arm is in position the investigator should begin verbally counting down from 10 while simultaneously counting down on his or her fingers in full view of the patient. Observe to detect any downward arm drift prior to the end of the 10 seconds. Downward movement that occurs directly after the investigator places the patient's arm in position should not be considered downward drift. Repeat this test for the opposite arm. This item should be scored for the right and left arm individually, denoted as item 5a and 5b.
0	No arm drift; the arm remains in the initial position for the full 10 seconds
1	Drift; the arm drifts to an intermediate position prior to the end of the full 10 seconds, but not at any point relies on a support
2	Limited effort against gravity; the arm is able to obtain the starting position, but drifts down from the initial position to a physical support prior to the end of the 10 seconds
3	No effort against gravity; the arm falls immediately after being helped to the initial position, however the patient is able to move the arm in some form (e.g. shoulder shrug)

Right and left motor function

4	No movement; patient has no ability to enact voluntary movement in this arm
Notes	✓ Default Coma Score: 8 ✓ Score should be recorded for each arm separately, resulting in a maximum potential score of 8. ✓ Motor Arm assessment should be skipped in the case of an amputee, however a note should be made in the scoring of the amputation.
Motor Leg	
score	How to perform: With the patient in the supine position, one leg is placed 30 degrees above horizontal. As soon as the patient's leg is in position the investigator should begin verbally counting down from 5 while simultaneously counting down on his or her fingers in full view of the patient. Observe any downward leg drift prior to the end of the 5 seconds. Downward movement that occurs directly after the investigator places the patient's leg in position should not be considered downward drift.
0	No leg drift; the leg remains in the initial position for the full 5 seconds
1	Drift; the leg drifts to an intermediate position prior to the end of the full 5 seconds, but at no point touches the bed for support
2	Limited effort against gravity; the leg is able to obtain the starting position, but drifts down from the initial position to a physical support prior to the end of the 5 seconds
3	No effort against gravity; the leg falls immediately after being helped to the initial position, however the patient is able to move the leg in some form (e.g. hip flex)
4	No movement; patient has no ability to enact voluntary movement in this leg
Notes	✓ Default Coma Score: 8 ✓ This is performed for each leg, indicating a maximum possible score of 8 ✓ Motor leg assessment should be skipped in the case of an amputee; however a note should be made in the score records
Limb Ataxia	
score	How to perform: The patient should be instructed to first touch his or her finger to the examiner's finger then move that finger back to his or her nose, repeat this movement 3-4 times for each hand. Next the patient should be instructed to move his or her heel up and down the

	shin of his or her opposite leg. This test should be repeated for the other leg as well.	
0	Normal coordination; smooth and accurate movement	
1	Ataxia present in 1 limb; rigid and inaccurate movement in one limb	
2	Ataxia present in 2 or more limbs: rigid and inaccurate movement in both limbs on one side	
Notes		
	✓ If significant weakness is present, score 0 ✓ If patient is unable to understand commands or move limbs, score is 0 ✓ Patient's eyes should remain open throughout this section	
Sensory		
score	How to perform: Sensory testing is performed via pinpricks in the proximal portion of all four limbs. While applying pinpricks, the investigator should ask whether or not the patient feels the pricks, and if he or she feels the pricks differently on one side when compared to the other side.[	
0	No evidence of sensory loss	
1	Mild-to-Moderate sensory loss; patient feels the pinprick, however he or she feels as if it is duller on one side	Left cortical function
2	Severe to total sensory loss on one side; patient is not aware he or she is being touched in all unilateral extremities	
Notes		
	✓ Default Coma Score: 2 ✓ The investigator should insure that the sensory loss being detected is a result of the stroke, and should therefore test multiple spots on the body. ✓ For patients unable to understand the instructions, the pinprick can be replaced by a noxious stimulus and the grimace can be judged to determine sensory score.	
Language		
score	How to perform: After completing the previous tests it is likely the investigator has gained an approximation of the patient's language skills; however it is important to confirm this measurement at this time. The stroke scale includes a picture of a picture of a scenario, a list of simple sentences, a figure of assorted random objects, and a list of words. The patient should be asked to explain the scenario depicted in the first figure. Next, he or she should read the list of sentences and name each of the objects depicted in the next figure. The scoring for this item should be based on both the results from the test performed in this item in	Left cortical function

	addition to the language skills demonstrated up to this point in the stroke scale.	
0	Normal; no obvious speech deficit	
1	Mild-to-moderate aphasia; detectable loss in fluency, however, the examiner should still be able to extract information from patient's speech	
2	Severe aphasia; all speech is fragmented, and examiner is unable to extract the figure's content from the patients speech.	
3	Unable to speak or understand speech	
Notes	✓ Default Coma Score: 3 ✓ Patients with visual loss should be asked to identify objects placed in his or her hands ✓ This is an exception to recording only the patients first attempt. In this item, the patient's best language skills should be recorded	
Speech		
score	How to perform: The patient is asked to read from the list of words provided with the stroke scale while the examiner observes the patient's articulation and clarity of speech.	Right motor function
0	Normal; clear and smooth speech	
1	Mild-to-moderate dysarthria; some slurring of speech, however the patient can be understood	
2	Severe dysarthria; speech is so slurred that he or she cannot be understood, or patients that cannot produce any speech	
Notes	✓ Default Coma Score:2 ✓ An intubated patient should not be rated on this item, instead make note of the situation in the scoring documents.	
Extinction and Inattention		
score	How to perform: a technique referred to as "double simultaneous stimulation". This is performed by having the patient close his or her eyes and asking him or her to identify the side on which they are being touched by the examiner. During this time the examiner is alternating between touching the patient on the right and left side. Next, the examiner touches the patient on both sides at the same time. This should be repeated on the patients face, arms, and legs. To test extinction in vision, the examiner should hold up one finger in front of each of the patient's eyes and ask the patient to determine which finger is wiggling	Left cortical function

	or if both are wiggling. The examiner should then alternate between wiggling each finger and wiggling both fingers at the same time.
0	Normal; patient correctly answers all questions
1	Inattention on one side in one modality; visual, tactile, auditory, or spatial
2	Hemi-inattention; does not recognize stimuli in more than one modality on the same side.
Notes	✓ Default Coma Score: 2 ✓ Patient with severe vision loss that correctly identifies all other stimulations scores a 0

INTERPTERION

Score	Stroke severity
0	No stroke symptoms
1-4	Minor stroke
5-15	Moderate stroke
16-20	Moderate to severe stroke
21-42	Severe stroke

Author's Biography

Mina Azer got his Master's degree in surgery in 2013. He has a great passion for science yielded in his current research and publications. Between 2004 and 2016 he shared in more than 70 different training delivered to more than 2000 trainees about various topics such as: reproductive health, surgical skills, and medical research. He worked at the Gastroenterology Surgical Center in Mansoura University, Egypt and at the Egyptian Liver Research Institute and Hospital. He is currently working at the Ubbo-Emmius Klinik in Norden, Germany.

www.ingramcontent.com/pod-product-compliance
Lightning Source LLC
Chambersburg PA
CBHW072149170526
45158CB00004BA/1569